how to reverse
facial ageing

the only things that work to rejuvenate your face

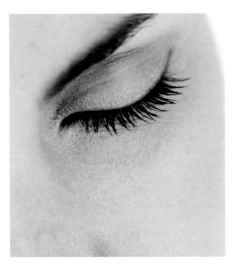

Doctor Brooke Seckel, MD
Clinical Professor of Surgery, Harvard Medical School

foulsham
LONDON • NEW YORK • TORONTO • SYDNEY

foulsham

The Publishing House, Bennetts Close, Cippenham, Slough,
Berkshire SL1 5AP, England

Foulsham books can be found in all good bookshops and direct from
www.foulsham.com

ISBN: 978-0-572-03288-3

First published 2005 in the US as *Save Your Face* by Peach Publications, Inc.,
Concord, Massachusetts

Cover photograph © Photolibrary

A CIP record for this book is available from the British Library

For more information about Dr Seckel, visit http://saveyourface.com

Printed in China through Colorcraft Ltd, Hong Kong

how to reverse
facial ageing

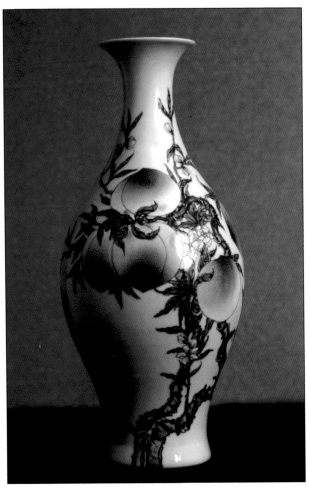

The peach: Chinese symbol of longevity.

In Chinese folklore, the peach is the symbol of longevity and immortality. The peach that grows on a special tree near the palace of Xiwangmu is considered a sacred fruit. Xiwangmu is queen of the immortals. The peach tree near her palace blooms every 3000 years and anyone who eats the fruit of this tree gains immortality. I love the beauty of the peach, but also present it to my readers in the hope that by reading this book they will partake of the peach and gain healthy longevity.

To Tommy and Laura

My joy and inspiration

Robert and Kathy

My friends

and

Martha

My guardian angel

Contents

Acknowledgements

Kathleen Burke not only provided superb illustrations for this book but also served as copy-editor, proof-reader, promoter, public relations officer and design consultant. More importantly, her close friendship and support throughout this entire project have played an essential role in its completion.

I express my deepest thanks to those who worked on the original, US edition of this book: Diane Bair, editor, Maria Fernanda Gamba, design and typesetting, Gilberto Gamba and Rick Chevalier, photo editing, and Melinda Steadman, manuscript preparation. Alvart Badalian of Arrow Graphics, Inc. worked on the cover and interior design for the second US edition.

I am also extremely grateful to Jan Nathan of Publishers Marketing Association and Dan Poynter of Para Publishing for their generous and invaluable mentoring during the production of this book. The entire staff at Independent Publishers Group are a gifted and dedicated group of professionals who have guided me successfully through the complex and challenging intricacies of marketing and distribution and have relieved me of one of publishing's most burdensome yet essential tasks.

I am blessed to be surrounded by a large group of professionals who provide daily support to me in my plastic surgery practice, both in my office and in the operating room. Without the kind and caring support of these individuals, the task of writing this book would have been much more difficult. Janice Ianone, Dawn O'Toole, Amy Defeo, Barbara Spracklin, Sheryl Scannel, Monique LeBlanc, Carolyn Newall, Mary Reed, Melinda Steadman, Amy Guertin, Ann Tobin, Ann Twomey, Christine Holman and Donna Cameron all are valued friends and associates whose kind support enables me to fulfil my multifaceted mission.

Finally, I am truly blessed and privileged to be a plastic surgeon for my many patients whose emotional feedback and trust have inspired me to continue looking for a better way to practise my profession. I am so grateful to them all.

With the second edition of the US version of this book, *Save Your Face*, I also started a new and exciting chapter in my life. I joined with Dr Bill Adams, who shares my vision of the future of plastic surgery and health and wellness in the twenty-first century. Dr Adams, one of Boston's finest plastic surgeons and founder of the Adams Center, has, like me, over 25 years of experience in this field. Together, with more than 50 years of experience between us, we have founded Mei, the medical spa of the future, in Boston, where, God willing, we will continue to innovate and bring happiness, good health and vigorous longevity to our wonderful patients.

Brooke R Seckel, MD

Photograph acknowledgements

With thanks to the following for the provision of additional photographs for this book:

© **Aesthetic Plastic Surgery:** page 81 top
© **AJ Photo:** page 167
© **Dr Alex Bartel:** pages 131, 132, 151
© **Anthory Blake Photo Library:** page 48
© **Lisa Bunin MD and Cutera™:** pages 98
© **Bruce M Friedman MD and Sciton™:** page 120
© **Ian Hooton:** pages 99, 101
© **Dr P Marazzi:** pages 52, 63, 85
© **Jason Pozner MD and Sciton™:** page 93
© **Retin-A™:** page 103
© **Bruce Russell MD and Cutera™:** pages 95 top, 96
© **Jo St Mart:** pages 48, 81 bottom, 86, 87, 92, 102, 104, 106, 109, 111, 115, 122, 124, 128, 134, 136, 146, 159, 160, 162, 164, 168, 170
© **Stockxpert:** pages 13, 14, 15, 16, 18, 20, 21, 22, 23, 24, 28, 31, 33, 37, 43, 44, 45, 46, 47, 51, 50, 53, 54, 55, 56, 57, 58, 60, 62, 64, 65, 67, 69, 70, 71, 72, 73, 74, 77, 79, 83, 88, 89, 90, 91, 137, 143, 149, 166

About the author

Dr Brooke R Seckel is a nationally and internationally recognised authority in plastic surgery and the treatment of facial ageing. He performs all types of cosmetic, facial and breast plastic surgery, but his special interest lies in the field of non-invasive and non-surgical therapies to correct and prevent facial ageing.

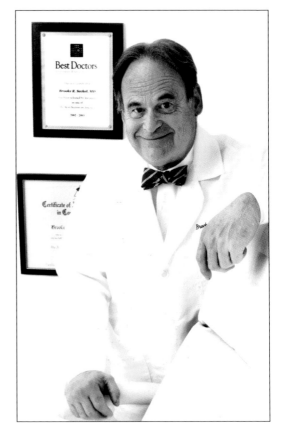

Dr Seckel founded and served as Director of the Lahey Center for Cosmetic and Laser Surgery in Lexington, Massachusetts, USA. He was the first chairman of the Department of Plastic Surgery at the Lahey Clinic in Burlington, Massachusetts, USA, a large multi-specialty group practice hospital in the Boston area.

He is certified by the **American Board of Plastic Surgery**, is a member of the **American Society of Plastic Surgeons**, the **American Society for Aesthetic Plastic Surgery** and the Boston Surgical Society, and an Assistant Clinical Professor of Surgery at Harvard Medical School, and was recently honoured by his peers by being voted one of the 'Best Doctors in America'.

Dr Seckel has published more than 100 scientific articles in the field of plastic surgery and authored the first book on cosmetic laser surgery, entitled *Aesthetic Laser Surgery*. He is also a board-certified neurologist and published *Facial Danger Zones*, a book devoted to teaching surgeons how to perform facial surgery safely without injuring the facial nerves.

Dr Seckel founded and served as Program Director of the Lahey Clinic Residency Program in Plastic Surgery. He has taught for many years that with advances in technology, plastic surgery is becoming less 'surgical' and more of a preventative discipline. The exciting advances in the field of anti-ageing medicine during the past 10 years prompted Dr Seckel to write this book, in which he presents a comprehensive preventative and therapeutic approach to the topic of **facial rejuvenation**.

Dr Seckel maintains an active plastic surgery practice on Newbury Street in the heart of Boston and in Peabody, Massachusetts, on Boston's North Shore. He is also Co-Director of Mei, Boston's leading-edge medical spa, where he specialises in the latest surgical and non-surgical facial rejuvenation techniques.

Dr Seckel resides in Concord, Massachusetts, and is the father of Laura and Tommy Seckel. In his spare time he enjoys sailing on Cape Cod, woodworking, building furniture, wooden boat restoration, restoring his antique home and jogging with his German Shepherd, Griffin.

Preface

I have been a physician for 35 years and a plastic surgeon for the past 24. Personally, there are few joys that match sharing the happiness and enthusiasm of my patients as they look into a mirror following plastic surgery. They see a face they remember, happily, from the past – a young face, a smiling face, a face looking ahead to the possibilities and dreams of the future. For me, plastic surgery is all about empowerment, about helping people realise their potential as human beings. Unfortunately, the effects of the ageing process, which has been going on since the day we were born, become dramatically visible on our faces long before our minds, bodies and spirits are willing to accept the notion that 'that's all there is'.

While some say we should 'grow old gracefully', my experience as a doctor (not to mention the recent explosion in the field of anti-ageing medicine) reveals that 'baby boomers' do not accept this irrelevant, out-dated concept.

Ageing transforms the face to create a tired, drawn look that belies the essence of the person inside. Contemporary Western society seems reluctant to acknowledge the fact that, behind an ageing face, is a vibrant person with the same visions, fantasies, goals, desires and needs of a younger person just starting adult life.

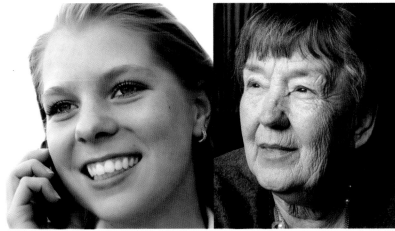

A tired, old face belies the energy and enthusiasm that remain inside.

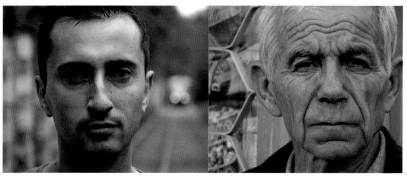

The effects of facial ageing can easily be seen by comparing a young face with an old one.

Sadly, for our society and for humankind, these changes are most apparent and most striking at a time in our lives when we have reached our greatest potential as human beings. In our middle years, we're enriched with the knowledge and wisdom gained through our experiences, so we approach the important events of life with a much more effective problem-solving strategy than we could when we were younger and less experienced. Our skills and our vitality, enhanced with our own strength and maturity, can improve the human experience for all.

What does looking younger have to do with such far-reaching and profound concepts?

There are at least two very important benefits to maintaining a youthful appearance. First, your appearance has a profound effect on your self-esteem, which is a major factor affecting your mood, enthusiasm and energy, factors that empower you to live a productive and fulfilling life. Second, for better or for worse, our youth-oriented, fast-paced, competitive culture promotes and values a youthful appearance over an old one.

This prejudice often impacts our careers and social lives in an inhibitory and harmful way. Loss of career opportunity and social relevance is particularly devastating to our sense of well-being, especially in a society in which traditional, long-term, mutually supportive relationships – such as marriage and long-term employment at one company – have ceased to be the norm.

I will not argue with those who tell me that my opinions and musings are vanity based, insecure and superficial. They are entitled to their view and may have it in peace. My opinions are my own, based on over 30 years of experience as a doctor, and are affirmed daily by the patients who make up my large and meaningful plastic surgical practice. My patients are wonderful, sane people who understand the issues of ageing and have the courage to resist feeling and looking older. They refuse to accept passively what fate has offered to previous generations. History will never describe our generation, the so-called 'baby boomer' generation, as passive!

My major concern regarding the current interest in the field of facial ageing is that technology is outpacing the ability of doctors to incorporate many of the new anti-ageing therapies safely into medical practice. Traditionally, a new medical therapy, like the polio vaccine, was tested and tried in the laboratory until it was proven to be safe and effective for human use. Only then was the new product made available to those doctors who possessed the knowledge and skills to use it safely for the benefit of patients.

The world of health care is a vastly different place today. Many manufacturers of medical equipment have made a conscious decision to focus their business on anti-ageing because they perceive the substantial potential for profit in this field. The same corporations have also learned the immense power of marketing.

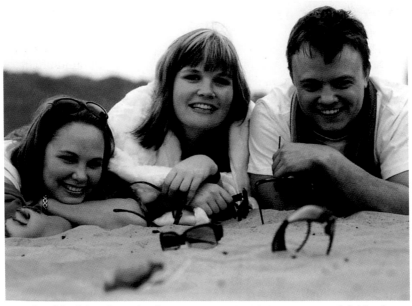

A healthy lifestyle is the first step in maintaining your youthful looks.

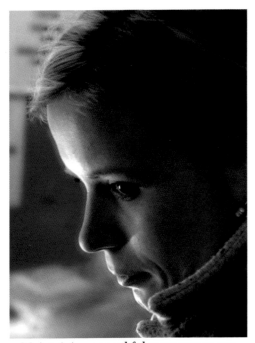

*Maintaining a youthful appearance can
have a profound effect on your self-esteem.*

Today, new anti-ageing technologies are seductively marketed directly to you, the consumer, not the doctor – often, in my opinion, before their effectiveness and safety have been proven. You, the potential patient, get excited by the, often unrealistic, marketing claims and demand these treatments from your doctor. The doctor is placed in a difficult position. He or she must pay the corporation for a hugely expensive laser to avoid being perceived as not up to date in the field and, worse, may lose patients to a doctor who already has the new machine.

Of course, when the therapies do not work, the truth will be known and the product will fail, but only after millions of pounds have changed hands from patient to doctor to corporation. If you doubt me, look on the Internet for advertisements for used medical lasers, machines available for a fraction of their original cost and described as 'like new'. Of course they are new. The machines did not deliver what was promised and were hardly used. It is to be hoped that no one was physically hurt during the short time the machines were in service.

Another alarming trend, particularly in the field of facial rejuvenation, is that many of the new anti-ageing therapies are being offered to patients by practitioners without medical degrees, in spas and other non-medical centres. This trend is partially due to the fact that many of the new therapies are non-invasive and appear so easy to perform that people assume that anyone can provide these treatments. Then there's the fact that the contemporary medical community has been slow to incorporate new anti-ageing therapies into current medical practice – even though, as this book documents, there is substantial credible scientific evidence to support many of the new therapies. Finally, non-physician entrepreneurs have discovered the immense financial potential of the field of facial anti-ageing and are eager to cash in on this bonanza without going to medical school and learning to treat patients in an appropriate and safe way.

Regardless of the circumstance, you, the patient, are exposed to unnecessary risks when you receive medical therapies from someone other than a knowledgeable and skilled doctor. What happens if some serious medical complication occurs in a spa and there is no doctor present? That's a frightening thought! I predict that the newly evolving 'medical spa' with physicians on staff will become the primary source for preventive medical care in the future. The model will be a true health-maintenance organisation helping patients prevent illness and live a healthy lifestyle.

In this book, I will present what I understand to be the truth about the causes, prevention and treatment of facial ageing. As a plastic surgeon, I know that we can successfully make your face look 20 or 30 years younger with surgery. The goal, however, is to prevent ageing of your face or, if that is not possible, to rejuvenate your face without harming you in the process.

Please be patient while reading this book. There is a great deal of technical information on the following pages, some of which is not

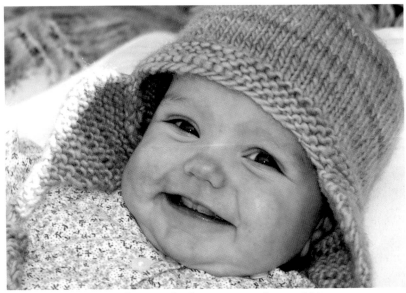

Stay closer to the face you were born with!

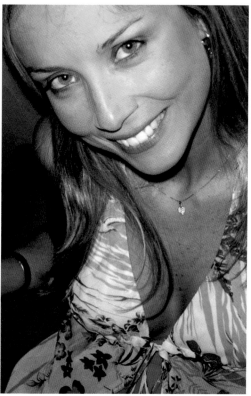

This book can help you become an educated consumer.

easy reading! But you need to know the facts if you are going to make informed choices. You need to understand the cause before you can go for the cure.

What you learn in this book will empower you to make the right choices and not be fooled by some advertisement that insults your intelligence by promising the fountain of youth, taking your money and leaving you unchanged or worse off than when you started. So relax, sit down with a cup of green tea and some soft music and start reading. It will take some time and effort on your part, but in the end you will be a very powerfully educated consumer in the new anti-ageing marketplace.

Why am I writing this book? First, I love to write. Second, I love to teach. Ultimately, it is because I get great joy from experiencing the beauty of restoration, whether I'm restoring a patient's face, my old wooden boat or my wonderful 160-year-old home.

Nothing makes me happier than seeing something showing signs of age brought back to gleaming brilliance once again, shining and new but with the glowing patina of depth and quality that only time and experience can produce.

Brooke R Seckel, MD
Concord, Massachusetts

1 *Is that my mother I see in the mirror?*

All of us reflect our heredity, and nowhere is that reflection more dramatic than in our facial appearance. The most common complaint of my 30–40-year-old patients when they first seek consultation for facial ageing is, 'I'm starting to look like my mother/father,' as the case may be. Of course they have always looked like Mum or Dad, but now they are starting to see wrinkles and other changes that make them resemble their 60-year-old or 70-year-old parent.

Look at the photograph below and try to understand exactly what it is that makes our faces look old. This picture is the first slide in my lecture about **plastic surgery** for facial ageing. It graphically

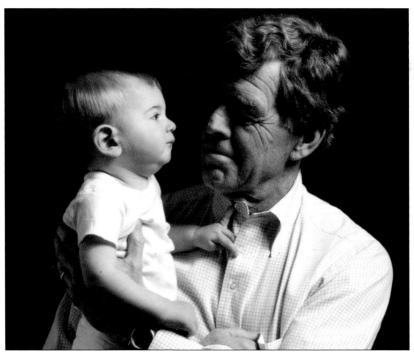

The effect of six decades of facial ageing on the faces we are born with.

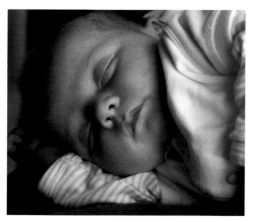

A baby's skin is plump, smooth and unblemished.

demonstrates the impact of six decades of ageing on the faces we are all born with.

The baby's skin is smooth, plump, unblemished, moist, radiant and firm, yet supple and elastic. If you gently pulled on the child's cheek and let go, the skin would snap back instantly, a quality we call **elasticity**. In contrast, the man's skin is rough and dry, with wrinkles and multiple blemishes – **brown spots** called **age spots**, and groups of small, dilated blood vessels called **telangiectasias**. There are also red spots with scaly, white, flaking skin over them called **actinic keratoses**, and these may eventually develop into **skin cancer**. The man's skin does not glow like that of the infant; the child's healthy radiance has been replaced by a sallow, dull, almost yellowish appearance.

These superficial changes are caused primarily by years of exposure to the sun and other harmful agents in the environment. Doctors refer to these superficial skin changes as Type I facial ageing changes. Type I facial ageing is most evident on the surface of the skin, the superficial skin layer called the **epidermis**.

The skin of the man is wrinkled and sagging, and hangs in folds on his face. If you grasped his skin with your thumb and index finger and let go, it would not snap back like the child's skin. Instead, it would take 5–10 seconds to go back to its original shape. This is **skin laxity**, the hallmark of aged facial skin. These changes are caused by age-associated damage to the deeper layers of

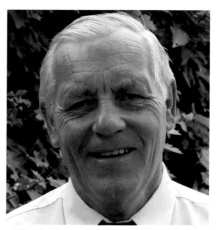

The hallmark of aged skin is the loss of the skin's elasticity.

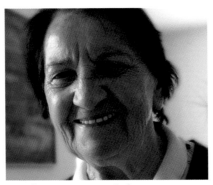

Changes around the eyes are particularly marked in an older face in response to the pull of the muscles of facial expression.

the skin, the **dermis**, and are called Type II facial ageing changes. Type II facial ageing changes are the result of our heredity, nutrition, exposure to the sun and other toxins, and lifestyle. The most important skin change that causes Type II facial ageing changes is the loss of the skin's elasticity. The cause of this **loss of elasticity** is damage to the **collagen** and **elastin**, two important structural proteins present in the dermis.

All modern facial rejuvenation therapies attempt to correct Type I and Type II facial ageing changes. Ageing changes in the face are complex and have an impact on different parts of the face in different ways at different times and in different people. Let's look at the diagram of the aged face in Figure 1.2 on page 19 and analyse the changes in each part.

The left side of this facial diagram shows the result of six or seven decades of sun damage and ageing. I like to analyse the face in thirds: the upper third (forehead and eyes), the middle third (cheeks and nose) and the lower third (mouth, jaw line and neck). Although the same ageing phenomenon is impacting all three areas, the results of facial ageing are different in each area and show up at different times in your life. The therapies that correct these ageing changes are different for each area. Understanding this concept will help you understand the correctional therapies discussed later in this book.

Eyelid changes are the earliest sign of facial ageing and are the first to occur in the upper third of the face. They

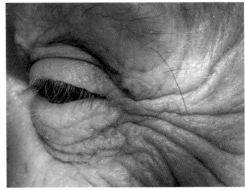

Crow's feet develop at the side of the eye, and eyelid bags on the lower eyelid.

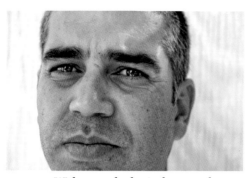

With age, dark circles can form beneath the eyes.

develop in almost all people in their thirties. The earliest changes are **wrinkles, crow's feet** at the side of the eyes, **worry lines** on the forehead, **frown lines** between the brows and **bunny lines** between the eyes. They are actually caused by the pull of our underlying **muscles of facial expression**, muscles that function to express our emotions.

Later, the upper eyelid skin begins to sag or droop over the eyelid fold (called the **supratarsal fold**) and eventually over the eyelashes themselves. This creates a tired look. The lower eyelid begins to show permanent lines or wrinkles associated with the same muscle pull that is causing the crow's feet.

Another lower eyelid change is puffiness or bagginess. This is caused by loss of elasticity of the skin and muscle of the eyelid. It allows the fat (which normally lies beneath the eyeball and supports it) to **herniate** (or push outwards) – a hernia is just a fancy term for a bulge. This change causes what is commonly referred to as **eyelid bags**. There are also textural skin changes in the eyelid that make the skin look old.

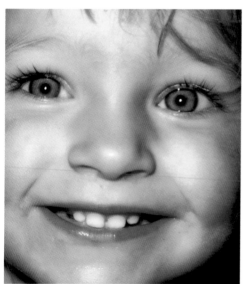

There are many non-surgical, **topical, laser** and other therapies that can remedy the superficial skin changes. However, once the deeper changes have occurred in the lower eyelid, plastic surgery is required to correct them. Claiming that a skin cream can significantly correct lax skin and bulging fat in the eyelid is, in my opinion, false advertising! Don't believe it.

The fat on a child's cheek is high up under the cheek bone.

Another very striking facial ageing change, which involves the upper third and middle third of the face, is called the **tear trough deformity**. It is that sad, oblique line that runs from just under the eyelid, starting at the nose and running out and down the very top of the cheek towards the ear. This is an advanced sign, which typically occurs in the late fifties to sixties, but it often begins in the late thirties or early forties as a **dark circle** or shadow beneath the eyelid. It is caused by the fact that your lower eyelid muscle is attached to the bone of your eye socket and therefore it can't fall downwards with the eyelid skin as the bulging fat pushes your eyelid out and down. As the cheek starts to fall, the area stays tethered to the bone, which creates an ever-increasing depression and shadow along the line.

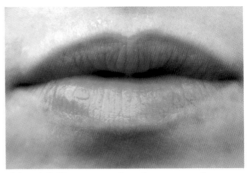

Lipstick lines can develop around the mouth in the thirties.

Early on, we call this change 'dark circles' or a 'tired look', but later it forms a deep line or trough into which your tears roll out to the side of your face and not straight down your cheek, as they did when you were a child – thus 'tear trough deformity'.

Now look at the eyebrows of the face in the diagram. The eyebrow has sagged or drooped down over the eye, especially the outer portion on the side of the face nearest the ear. This phenomenon is called **brow ptosis** and is caused not only by loss of elasticity of the skin, but also by the sagging of fat that lies beneath the eyebrow.

There are several major facial ageing events occurring in the middle of the face that create an aged appearance. The most profound is the sagging of the cheek, which produces the fold of skin hanging down around the mouth called the **nasal–labial fold**. This ageing change is caused by two things: laxity, or the loss of elasticity of the skin and underlying structures of the face (which allows gravity to pull the skin down), and the fall of the **malar fat pad**, or cheek fat pad.

As a child, this pad of fat under the cheek skin is attached high up on your cheekbone, just under the eyes. Remember those chubby cheeks that all the grown-ups liked to pinch? Look at your children; they have nice, full cheeks high on their faces. As we age, the malar fat pad descends into the middle of the cheek. Making things worse are your smile muscles. Look in the mirror and smile; do you see the **smile line**? It is caused by muscles that pull on the corners of your mouth, drawing it up and out to the sides when you smile. The smile line runs from the corner of your nose to the corner of your mouth. Notice how the cheek hangs over this line? The combination of the loss of elasticity (which allows the skin to sag), the downward fall of the malar fat pad and years of smiling creates the deep smile line with folds of skin hanging over it, which we call the **nasal–labial fold line**. The action of the smile muscles also creates wrinkles in the cheek, which become permanent as the skin ages. Also notice that as the malar fat pad has dropped, forming the nasal–labial fold, there is a facial depression where it used to be. This depression contributes to the tear trough deformity.

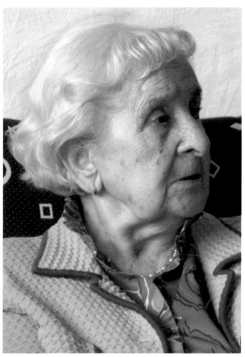

The loosening of the muscles under the chin causes the neck skin to become loose.

Facial ageing has a profound effect on the lower third of the face. Vertical wrinkles, called **lipstick lines**, develop around the lips fairly early, often in the thirties. Smoking horribly accentuates these lines. If you don't smoke, you may never get them, or they will be smaller and less significant. The upper lip also sags due to loss of elasticity and **atrophy** (wasting away) of normal fat inside the lip. As a result, the lip becomes longer. Did you ever hear the expression 'long in the tooth' in reference to old people? The pink part of your upper lip, the 'Cupid's bow', becomes thinner and turns downwards and inwards, and the corners of the mouth turn down. The most common complaint I hear is, 'People think I am angry or mean and I am not.' This is especially true when deep frown lines and ageing changes around the mouth are present in the same face. The sagging of the cheek, which causes the nasal–labial fold, also causes the skin to fall down over the corner of the mouth and chin to form **marionette lines**. The chin also droops in some people, usually only in their late fifties or sixties, and it can be distressing to those who experience it. The horrible term 'witch's chin' is used to describe it.

The descent of the facial skin also causes sagging along the jaw line, creating **jowls**. As the neck ages, the neck skin becomes lax and falls into folds below the chin, referred to as **turkey wattle**. Frequently, there are prominent bands on the neck, called **platysmal bands** because they are caused by the pull and laxity of the two platysma muscles underneath the chin. These muscles act like cords, pulling the skin folds down along two lines running from under the chin to the middle of the neck.

These changes are what many people can expect to see after 70 years of facial ageing if they do not take steps to prevent them. However, the severity of ageing in the face varies, depending on your genetic make-up and how well you take care of yourself. Don't expect face creams to correct these major structural changes, even though this concept is often promoted in the media. Those who fall for this idea do not understand the complex anatomical changes that occur in the ageing face.

Fortunately, you are reading this book, so you won't be misled. You obviously do not want to end up like the person in Figure 1.2 or you would not have bought the book! I don't want you to end up like that either. In Chapter 2, we take a close-up look at what causes these distressing changes to occur in our faces, but first let's summarise in Table 1.1 what we have learned so far.

The age ranges in Table 1.1 are generalisations. People with Type I and Type II skin, redheads and fair blondes (see Table 3.1 in Chapter 3 for **skin types**) will age earlier, at the lower end of the age range. Darker-skinned patients will age later. Smokers, drinkers and people with unhealthy lifestyles will age and develop facial wrinkles much earlier.

Table 1.1 Changes that occur in the skin with age

Ageing change	When first seen	Cause	Type	Correctable?
Brown spots; broken blood vessels; dry, rough skin	28–30 years	Sun and other toxic damage to superficial skin, the epidermis	Type I	Yes
Frown lines	28–30 years	Pull of facial muscle	Type II	Yes
Worry lines	28–30 years	Pull of facial muscle	Type II	Yes
Crow's feet	28–30 years	Pull of facial muscle	Type II	Yes
Lipstick lines	30–40 years	Atrophy of fat; pursing of muscle of lip; smoking	Type II	Yes
Nasal–labial fold lines	30–40 years	Skin laxity; pull of smile muscle	Type II	Partial correction
Neck laxity; early turkey wattle	30–40 years	Skin laxity	Type II	Yes
Jowling	40–50 years	Skin laxity	Type II	Yes
Tear trough deformity	50–60 years	Skin laxity; descent of malar fat pad	Type II	Partial correction
Marionette lines	50–60 years	Skin laxity; pull of smile muscle	Type II	Partial correction

2 Through the microscope

The skin is the body's largest organ, and one of the most important. We cannot live without skin, which is a major reason why extensive body burns are so often disabling or fatal. The skin is a living organ, just like your heart, lungs, liver, stomach and intestines. It protects you from the sun and your environment. It holds your vital essence inside. It keeps you hydrated, is the first line of defence against toxins and bacteria, and plays a crucial role in your immune system, which is your strategic defence system against all foreign invaders. The skin provides wound healing, controls heat loss, produces vitamin D for bone health and protects against some cancers. Skin produces the skin oil **sebum**, which keeps it moist, healthy and protected.

Let's look through a microscope at a section of healthy, normal, young skin, magnified about 100 times (Figure 2.1).

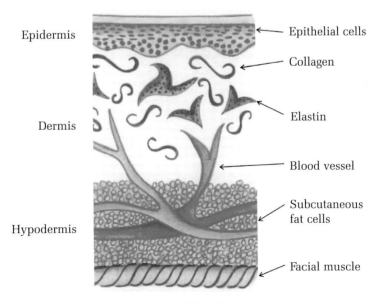

Figure 2.1 Healthy skin

The **cells** of the outer layer of the skin, the epidermis, are called **epithelial cells**. These cells, millions of them, are what you see on the surface of your face. The outer skin surface actually consists of many layers of epithelial cells. New cells are formed in the deeper layers every day and then grow upwards to replace the damaged, old cells on the surface.

One reason why all anti-ageing, beauty and wrinkle therapies include **exfoliation** (removing the top layer of damaged epithelial cells) is that the deeper, newer, plumper, healthier cells look better, and give the skin a fresh glow. It is important to understand that the epithelium is a living layer. As such, it can regenerate, restore and renew itself, which means that you can take steps to prevent and correct the ageing changes that affect it. We'll discuss this in detail later.

The second, deeper layer of the skin, the dermis, is where some of the most striking and important changes occur with facial ageing, which lead to the loss of elasticity discussed earlier. That loss of elasticity, you'll recall, is what causes wrinkling and sagging of the face. The dermis is the pink portion of your skin you see when you scrape the outer layer or when you injure your knee or hand. It will bleed when injured deeply. The dermis attaches your skin to your body and provides vital structural support, oxygen and nutrients to the epidermis, keeping the outer skin alive.

Three major components of the dermis, which are crucial to the ageing process, are collagen, elastin and **hyaluronic acid**. Collagen is a protein produced by a special cell called the **fibroblast**. Elastin is a special type of collagen that gives your skin elasticity – acting rather like a

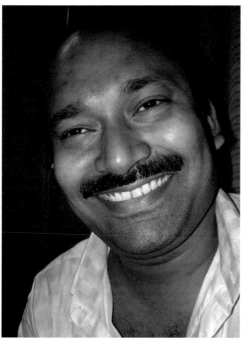

The plumping effect of fat contributes to a healthy skin appearance.

rubber band holding your skin on your face. When the elastin is damaged or weakened, your face becomes lax or loose, develops wrinkles and sags.

Hyaluronic acid, known as HA, is a complex substance called a mucopolysaccharide. It is present in the dermis and epidermis, surrounding and supporting all the cells, including the collagen. Most importantly, it helps maintain the moisture content of the dermis and the epidermis.

Some of the most striking and important changes that occur with facial ageing (and lead to the loss of elasticity and wrinkling discussed in Chapter 1) take place in the dermis. Underneath the dermis is the subcutaneous (under the skin) fat, which supports and protects the skin, nerves, blood vessels, muscles and other vital structures. It is a normal component of the skin from the time of birth. Fat functions when the skin is bumped, pressed or pushed. Push on the skin of your cheek and you will see that the skin virtually slides over the fat, which prevents it tearing. The plumping or filling effect of fat also contributes to a healthy skin appearance. Have you ever noticed how some overweight people do not have wrinkles? So resist the impulse to have your fat sucked out!

Now that you understand the structure of normal healthy skin, let's explore some of the changes that occur as we age and that result in the appearance of the older man in the picture in Chapter 1.

Look at Figure 2.2, the aged skin, and notice the striking changes. The vital health-sustaining functions of the skin decline to about one-third or two-thirds of their normal level by the eighth decade.[1] The skin is thinner, due to atrophy (wasting away) of the epidermis, the dermis and the underlying fat. The epidermal cells are less plump and less healthy looking and undergo many changes, which can ultimately lead to skin cancer. The number of **pigment cells** increases in an attempt to protect the skin from the damaging effect of the sun, resulting in brown age spots on the face. With thinning of the skin, the blood vessels begin to show through it as telangiectasias (small dilated blood vessels), which are most noticeable at an early stage around the nose and cheeks. Eventually, the thinning of the skin and the overgrowth of blood vessels (caused by **free-radical** damage) produce a pink or red flush on the cheeks and nose, a condition called **rosacea**. Skin pores are more prominent and enlarge as the supporting collagen around them disappears. These superficial changes are the Type I facial ageing changes.

Elastosis

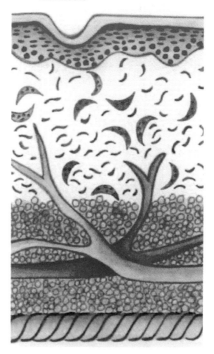

Figure 2.2 In sun-damaged skin, the healthy collagen and elastin of the dermis are replaced by fragmented elastin and scar tissue.

The most striking ageing changes take place in the dermis. Over time, collagen and elastin are destroyed and the number of deeper, larger blood vessels, oil glands, hair follicles and fibroblasts (recall that they make new collagen) in the dermis decreases. The dermis thins by 20 per cent as we age.[2] The effects of ageing are most profound on the elastin, which, you'll recall, is the rubber band-like fibre that holds our skin tight. These fibres are broken and fragmented and lose their ability to give elasticity to our skin. The loss of elasticity allows the skin to sag and wrinkle, and folds form in the face.

Under the microscope, the hallmark of sun-damaged, aged skin is **solar** (sun) **elastosis**, seen as a large accumulation of damaged elastin piled up in the dermis, replacing the healthy pink collagen apparent in normal skin. Remember, this phenomenon causes our facial skin to sag and wrinkle. Almost all modern facial anti-ageing treatments – from **skinceuticals** to lasers, **intense pulsed light** (IPL),

Thermage™, Titan™, **skin peels** and **microdermabrasion** – attempt to restore new, healthier collagen. These treatments are discussed in later chapters.

Hyaluronic acid, the moisturising matrix supporting the dermis and epidermis, is also lost with ageing. HA allows nutrients to reach the skin cells and also holds water, moisturises the skin and helps keeps it soft and supple. By the age of 50, there is a 50 percent reduction in the HA content of the skin.[3] That is huge. No wonder people complain of dry skin at 50!

In addition, the underlying subcutaneous fat atrophies, resulting in the loss of its plumping and protective effect on your skin. The muscles beneath your facial skin, which give you facial expression, also ultimately atrophy, but not before they have done their damage. The muscles of facial expression – around your eyes, the smile muscle in the cheek, and those around your mouth – continually contract and pull on your skin throughout your life. The result: those delightful lines of facial expression, including worry lines, frown lies, bunny lines, crow's feet, smile lines and lipstick lines. The facial ageing changes that occur as a result of these deeper dermal changes are called Type II facial ageing changes.

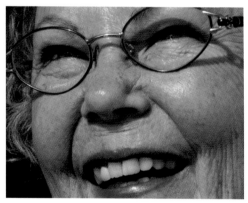

The lines of facial expression are caused by changes deep in the skin.

Table 2.1 overleaf summarises what we have learned in this chapter.

Table 2.1 The effects of the different types of facial ageing changes

Type of ageing changes	Location of damage	What we see
Type I	Epidermis vessels	Dry skin, brown spots, broken blood vessels, large pores
Type II	Dermis, subcutaneous fat	Wrinkles, skin laxity, lines of facial expression

References

1. Venna, S.S. and Gilchrest, B.A. Skin ageing and photo-ageing. *Skin & Ageing* 12:56, 2004.
2. Yaar, M. and Gilchrest, B.A. Ageing of skin. In I.M. Freidberg, A.Z. Eisen, K. Wolff et al. (eds), *Dermatology in General Medicine*. New York: McGraw-Hill, 1999, p. 1697.
3. Meschino, J.P. *The Wrinkle Free Zone*. North Bergen, NJ: Basic Health Publications, 2004, p. 49.

3 Ageing – cellular suicide!

Harsh, but true. We age because the cells of our bodies die or are killed by toxins or something harmful we do to them. There are two major types of ageing that occur in the cells that constitute your face and in all of the tissues and organs in your body. The first type is **intrinsic ageing** (from the inside). This results from a combination of your genetic (inherited) ageing pattern and your dietary and lifestyle factors, which have a profound influence on your rate and severity of ageing. Second is **extrinsic ageing** (from the outside), which is caused by toxic environmental and other harmful factors that damage the health of your skin and accelerate facial ageing.

Established science[1, 2] tells us that about 80 per cent of skin ageing is intrinsic and 20 per cent extrinsic. In the sections below we discuss the specific factors that initiate or cause these harmful ageing changes in your skin and body. I know that this is dry reading, but what you learn here will help you understand what causes facial ageing, and if you understand that, you can objectively evaluate the proposed cures and decide for yourself if they are realistic and if they make sense to you.

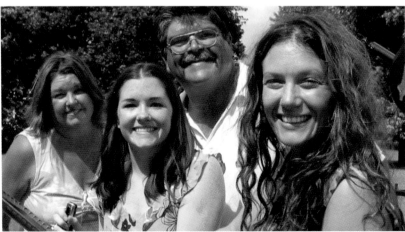

Anti-ageing strategies can help you live a longer and healthier life.

More importantly, the anti-ageing therapies we'll discuss will save your face, and they may also save your life. These anti-ageing strategies may help you live longer and may lessen your risk of cancer, heart disease and many other diseases that can end your life prematurely.

Ageing is a very complex, multifaceted problem. There is no one theory that is agreed upon by all doctors and scientists. The literature on ageing is voluminous, highly technical and hard to understand. I will try to distil a great deal of information in a simplified, comprehensible way, which will, I hope, make sense to you and enable you to make some very important decisions about your health. Be patient and read on.

Intrinsic ageing

The cell – the basic building block of life

Our bodies are made up of billions of tiny cells. In Chapter 2, you saw pictures of the cells of the outer layer of the skin, the epithelial cells. Every structure in the body is made up of specialised cells – muscles, bones, brain, gut, liver and all of our life-giving tissues. When enough of these cells die, we die! A **heart attack** kills the cells of the heart, so that it can no longer function to pump blood to the brain and other parts of the body, and we die. Some of our body parts are more important than others. We can live after losing a leg or an eye, but not without a functioning heart.

When we are born, if we do not have a birth defect, the cells of our bodies are healthy and function properly, a state we call 'good health' (Figure 3.1). To stay healthy and grow, each of our cells must be able

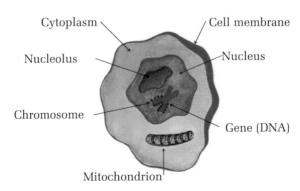

Figure 3.1 A healthy cell, the basic structural unit of all life.

to divide into two new cells, over and over again. This is a vital process. After we become adults, the daily work of living, digesting food, resisting infection, walking, working – virtually everything we do – requires the cells of our bodies to work very hard to keep us alive. Eventually, our cells wear out, so the old cells must divide to create new cells to enable our bodies to continue to function.

However, our cells cannot go on dividing forever. In fact, most cells are programmed at birth to divide only 70 times during the course of our lives.[3] Eventually, they stop dividing and die and no new cells are produced, and when enough of our vital, life-sustaining cells no longer function, we die. Cell death is, in essence, intrinsic ageing.

Why does this happen to our cells? Why can't they divide forever and allow us to go on living forever? It is God's will, perhaps. Theorists opine that once we have passed our childbearing years, we have outlived our usefulness to the planet, since our essential role is to produce offspring and renew life on the Earth. Following this line of thinking, once this task is accomplished, we must age and die so that there will be adequate resources, such as food and space, for new generations of humans.

Another important reason that our cells are not allowed to divide indefinitely and uncontrollably is that uncontrolled cell division equals cancer. A cancer is basically a mass of rapidly and uncontrollably dividing cells. The uncontrolled division of breast cells is breast cancer; the uncontrolled division of colon cells is colon cancer, and so on. Thus, our bodies must be able to control cell division to avoid cancer developing in our organs. The key to discovering a cure for cancer is discovering how to turn off this uncontrolled cell division and kill the cancer by making its cells grow old.

Inside your cells – DNA and your genetic heritage

DNA is a protein that makes up our **genes**, tiny packets of information that are attached to **chromosomes** (Figure 3.2).

Chromosomes reside in the centre of cells, in the nucleus. Every time our cells divide, the chromosomes divide, providing a complete set of genes and DNA to each of the two new cells. The DNA present in your genes spells out specific messages or detailed instructions to your cells to tell them what to do, what to make and when to divide.

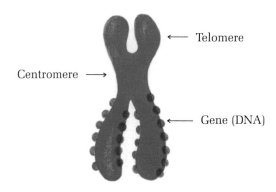

Figure 3.2 A healthy chromosome with attached genes consisting of DNA.

DNA is the basic structure that controls all of the functions of every cell in our bodies. Thus, our DNA is the ultimate factor that determines when and how we age. Have you noticed how some people look young for their age? I have seen people in their fifties who look as though they are 30 years old, and I am a professional at evaluating facial ageing! Some 40-year-old people have grey hair, deep wrinkles and sagging skin, whereas others of the same age may have dark hair and smooth, moist skin, with no wrinkles or laxity. The difference between these individuals is due to the difference in their DNA. (Some would call it luck!)

There are six basic types of skin and each one is determined by heredity. See Table 3.1 and identify your skin type.

Table 3.1 Hereditary skin types

Skin/hair/ eye colour	Skin type	Tendency to burn	Tendency to tan	Tendency to age	Type of ageing changes
White/red/blue	Type I	Always	Never	Early and severe	Types I and II
White/blonde/ blue or brown	Type II	Usually	Sometimes	Early	Types I and II
White/brown/ dark brown	Type III	Usually	Usually	Later	Type II
Brown to black/ black/brown	Type IV –VI	Never	Always	Very much later	Type II

The information that controls the type of skin we have is carried in the DNA in our genes on the chromosomes that we inherit from our parents.

Understanding your skin type is important because different skin types age very differently. Your inherited DNA, plus your nutrition, lifestyle and exposure to toxins, determine not only how you look and how your skin ages, but also how the rest of your body ages. We now know that heart disease, cancer and many of the diseases that lead to premature ageing, disability and death are influenced by our heredity.

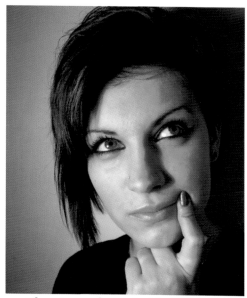

There's an element of luck – in our DNA – that influences how well we age.

But do not despair: we can now do a great deal to forestall or prevent these genetic catastrophes by lifestyle and nutritional modifications (see Chapter 4). The ultimate goal of the **Human Genome Project** is to work out how to modify genes to stop or prevent diseases that cause human suffering and death.

The telomere – your biological ageing clock

A **telomere** is a small DNA tail that is attached to every chromosome (see Figure 3.2) and that protects the chromosome during cell division. When cells divide, they do so only after the chromosomes divide, and it is important that each new cell has all the genes necessary for health and proper functioning. There is a risk during the cell division process that the chromosomes can be damaged and lose some of the genes. If genes and the crucial DNA they contain are lost, the new cells cannot function normally and may die or, worse, create abnormal products that can cause harm. The telomere protects the end of the chromosome by keeping it together and preventing the loss of any genes as it divides. This is a very important function.

The telomere loses some of its DNA each time the cell divides, and it therefore keeps getting shorter. Some scientists theorise that when our telomeres are shortened too much or are lost, the cells die – and so do we. Research has also identified short telomeres in people with short life spans, but some animals with longer telomeres than humans have shorter life spans than humans, so we do not have all the answers yet.

Scientists have discovered an enzyme called **telomerase**, which can prevent telomeres from getting shorter when the cell divides. Researchers theorise that if telomerase can be used to prevent shortening of the telomere, cell division can go on indefinitely and therefore we, and our cells, can become immortal. The problem is that unrestrained or immortal cell division is cancer, and in fact telomerase may well play a role in cancer cell growth. Some scientists hope that blocking telomerase may be a way to kill cancer cells and cure cancer. This field is very exciting, and future discoveries will undoubtedly have an impact on both cancer and ageing research. If you want to read more about telomeres, visit http://gslc.genetics.utah.edu/features/telomeres/.

Free radicals destroy our cells and DNA and cause inflammation and facial ageing

If you have not heard about free radicals by now, you certainly will very soon. If you want to 'save your face' and already take **antioxidant vitamins** every morning, you are halfway there. Free radicals have a major impact on facial ageing, and this topic is so important and the discovery of relevant new therapies is occurring so rapidly that I think it is essential to have a good understanding of the subject.

The cells in our bodies are made up of complex **molecules**, and molecules are made up of **atoms**. The atom, the basic sub-microscopic unit of which we are made, has positive (+) electrical charges called **protons** on the inside and negative (–) electrical charges called **electrons** on the outside. The electrons spin around the protons in the centre of the atom like a satellite spins around the Earth, held in orbit by the gravitational pull of the Earth.

The negatively charged electrons are kept close to the atom by the pull of the opposite, positive, charge of the protons. This is similar to the way opposite ends of two magnets are attracted and attach to each other (Figure 3.3).

The two opposite charges together are in balance and there is no overall charge, and therefore no effect, on the rest of the cell. The electrons that exert one negative charge actually consist of two small spinning electrons, and there is a substantial amount of energy holding this electron pair in orbit around the proton in the centre of the atom. These paired charges – that is, the proton (+) and electron (–) pair – keep the atom stable (Figure 3.3).

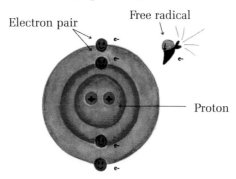

Figure 3.3 An atom with stable electrons in orbit.

A free radical is formed when some outside force steals or knocks one of the paired electrons away from its stable orbit around the atom (Figure 3.4).

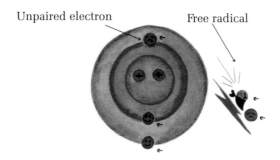

Figure 3.4 An unstable atom becomes a free radical.

The result? The atom that has lost the electron becomes very unstable. It now has an unpaired electron in the outer orbit, so it is now a free radical. It creates havoc in the cells by searching around and trying to steal a negatively charged electron away from another stable atom that has paired electrons in the outer orbit. The free-radical scientists (in reality, most of them are very tame, but they like the name) often call these free radicals 'promiscuous'. On a cellular level, this is a very high-energy process, not unlike a hurricane or an earthquake, and a great deal of damage is done in your cells when free radicals are formed. This damage occurs in two ways.

1. Free radicals damage the **cell membrane**, the 'shell' that encloses the contents of the cell. This damage can kill the cell or, if it is not fatal, can have an impact on the ability of the cell to carry out important life-sustaining functions (Figure 3.5).

2. When free radicals attack, they damage the DNA. This can destroy the genes that control the cells' vital functions (Figure 3.6).

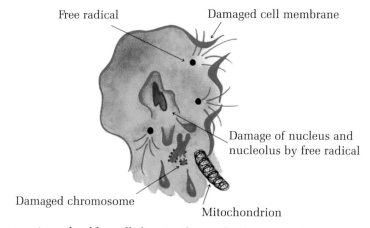

Free radical

Damaged cell membrane

Damage of nucleus and nucleolus by free radical

Damaged chromosome

Mitochondrion

Figure 3.5 An unhealthy cell showing free-radical damage to the cell wall and DNA (genes) on a chromosome.

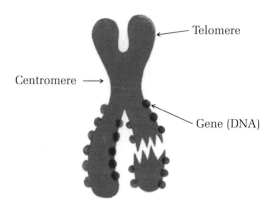

Telomere

Centromere →

Gene (DNA)

Figure 3.6 An unhealthy chromosome showing damage by free radicals.

Where do free radicals come from? Believe it or not, most of the free radicals in our bodies come from the oxygen we breathe. Oxygen is used by the **mitochondria**, which are small structures in our cells that convert our food into energy (Figure 3.7).

During this process, a great number of free radicals are produced (Figure 3.8).

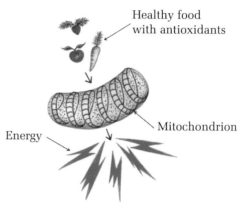

Figure 3.7 Healthy mitochondria in the cell convert our food to energy.

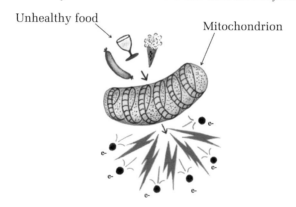

Figure 3.8 An unhealthy mitochondrion. Mitochondria also produce free radicals during the energy production process, especially when unhealthy foods are ingested.

Fortunately, our bodies have built-in protective mechanisms called **free-radical scavengers** that clean up these free radicals before they can do harm. The free-radical scavengers require the presence of the antioxidant vitamins A, C and E (and many others) in appropriate amounts for this protective system to work. When we do not have adequate amounts of these important vitamins or we are subjected to too many free radicals, the system is overloaded, damage occurs and our cells are either destroyed or no longer function normally.

In summary, free radicals are formed as follows.

❦ We eat food.

❦ Food is broken down and the nutrients go into our cells and into the mitochondria.

❦ The mitochondria take the food, add oxygen and make energy to keep us alive.

❦ Energy production produces atoms with good, paired electrons, but also produces some free radicals.

❦ These free radicals damage the cell membrane and DNA. The result: your cells die or are altered in such a way that they produce very harmful products.[4]

Inflammation – the basic cause of facial ageing

When our DNA and cell membranes are injured by free radicals (or anything else for that matter), the damaged cell membranes release a toxic substance called **arachidonic acid**. The damaged DNA also causes the release of **cytokines**, the chemical messengers that tell the rest of the body that damage has occurred. Both of these substances initiate a process called **inflammation**.

Inflammation is the response of the cells of the body to injury, cell damage or death, which can be caused by trauma, toxins, bacteria, viruses or other foreign invaders as well as by free radicals. Inflammation is the attempt by the body to stop and isolate the damage and keep it from spreading.

The signals put out by the damaged cells, carried by cytokines, tell the blood to send in **macrophages**. Macrophages are specialised blood cells that ingest the damaged cells and remove them from the area. The macrophages then take the damaged cells back to the bloodstream and eventually to the lymph nodes, from where they are removed from the body.

Inflammation is a very important, life-saving process. It protects us from harmful bacterial infection, helps heal our wounds and removes dead or damaged cells from our bodies.

The problem is that inflammation also produces some damaging chemicals and events inside our bodies that contribute to facial ageing. Worse, inflammation can be turned against us in a way that results in an **autoimmune response**. An autoimmune response occurs when inflammation attacks and destroys the normal body cells. This is disastrous, and scientists are discovering that many of the diseases we attribute to old age, such as

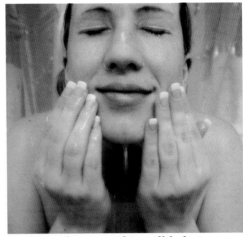

Looking after your skin will help to keep it healthy.

heart disease, some cancers and Alzheimer's disease, may in fact be caused by our own inflammatory processes turned against us.

Once inflammation has been initiated by the cytokines, it triggers a series of chain reactions. The macrophages not only clean up the damaged cells, but also send messages to cause other cells, called **mast cells**, to release **histamine**, a substance that dilates the blood vessels. Histamine makes the blood vessels leaky, and the injured site becomes filled with fluid and blood. This is why an injured site on the body becomes red and swollen. One example of inflammation that is very relevant with regard to facial ageing is sunburn.

Prolonged or severe inflammation is very destructive to the cells and tissues that the body is trying to protect and heal. Once the dead cells and debris are cleaned up, the macrophages convert to fibroblasts, which, you'll recall, are the cells that produce collagen. The collagen produced during inflammation forms a **scar**. When free radicals cause damage to your cells and produce inflammation in your skin, your healthy collagen is destroyed, and the scar collagen functions poorly. The result is wrinkles and damaged, sagging skin.

Hormones – internal modulators of cell function

Hormones are substances secreted by the glands of the body: the pituitary gland in the brain, the thyroid gland in the neck, the pancreas near the stomach, and the adrenal gland above each kidney. These hormones serve vital, life-giving roles by stimulating the cells of the body to carry out the important functions that keep us alive. As we age, the levels of various hormones decline, as do cellular functions that are dependent on these hormones. These events have a major impact on facial ageing.

It is important to understand that **hormone replacement therapies** should be used only when clinically significant deficiencies exist. Hormone replacement should only be carried out under the supervision of a doctor.

Cortisol – the stress hormone

Elevated levels of the adrenal hormone **cortisol** have a dramatic and profound ageing effect on the cells of the face and body. When you are stressed, you worry, and we have already discussed the effects of worry lines on the face. More importantly, cortisol is very damaging to the cells that make up the facial skin and other important organs

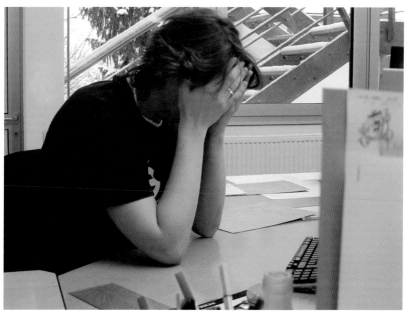

Stress leads to increased levels of the hormone cortisol, which can have a dramatic impact on your appearance.

in the body. Cortisol is released by the adrenal glands when you are in danger and need to go on 'high alert' to protect yourself. It speeds up your heart, pushes blood into your muscles, increases the energy produced by your muscle cells, and basically prepares you for 'fight or flight'. The problem is that if you stay pumped up like this all the time, you exhaust the cells of your body.

The stress of living in contemporary society, overextending ourselves and living under immense time pressure causes our adrenal glands to produce excess

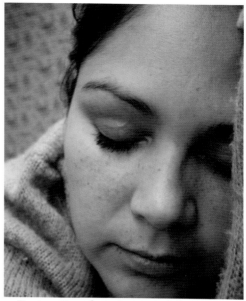

Restorative sleep is essential to good looks and good health.

cortisol. Prolonged, excessively high cortisol levels worsen intrinsic facial ageing changes by directly damaging collagen. They disturb the ability of the pancreatic hormone **insulin** to metabolise sugar and fats properly, and can deplete the body's immune system, all of which can lead to inflammation.[3]

Oestrogen, progesterone and testosterone – the sex hormones

The sex hormones have profound effects on facial ageing. During **menopause**, there is a 90 per cent decrease in **oestrogen** levels and a 66 per cent decrease in progesterone, both of which cause thinning and dryness of the skin.[5] In male **andropause**, **testosterone** levels drop by 50 per cent,[6] which not only thins the skin, but also reduces muscle mass.

Human growth hormone

Produced by the pituitary gland, **human growth hormone** (hGH) also decreases during ageing. Replacement therapy has been associated with restoration of muscle mass, energy and libido and improvement in skin ageing changes. However, the only regimen that has been proved to work is by injection. Most oral forms, which are supposed to stimulate the pituitary gland to make more hGH, are not effective.

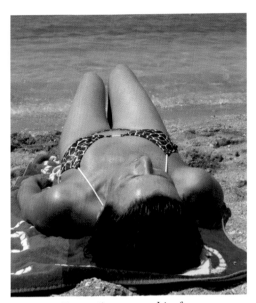

Protecting your skin from sun damage is absolutely essential.

More importantly, I'm afraid to take hGH injections for a very key reason: hGH works by making cells in the body divide to create brand new cells. Remember, cells that divide too much also cause cancer. Intelligent medical opinion holds that not enough is known about hGH cell-dividing stimulation to be sure that it is safe. Your doctor should check your hGH level. If it is low, consider replacement therapy. If it is normal, I do not recommend having hGH replacement. Personally, I would rather have wrinkles than cancer any day!

Melatonin – the anti-ageing hormone

Melatonin, a hormone secreted by the pineal gland in the brain, is called the anti-ageing hormone. It is a powerful **antioxidant** and free-radical scavenger and is also reported to be involved in supporting the immune system and thus fighting inflammation.[7, 8] It also plays an important role in our sleep/wake cycles, which enable us to rest and our body to restore itself. Melatonin is depleted by the stress hormone cortisol.

Extrinsic ageing

Traditionally, discussions of extrinsic ageing focused only on the damage caused by **ultraviolet** (UV) **light** from the rays of the sun on the skin. However, as our knowledge of the ageing process has expanded, we have become aware of a host of other factors that we take into our bodies that also cause significant free-radical damage and contribute to the ageing process. I'm including some of these factors in the extrinsic ageing category because we choose whether or not we take them into our bodies.

Sunlight

The UV wavelengths of the sun's rays have a dramatic, destructive ageing effect on the skin, especially if you are a fair-skinned Type I or Type II skin type. The UV radiation damages the epithelial cells, destroys collagen and elastin and is a major cause of the Type I skin changes discussed in Chapter 2. There is much evidence that the ageing effect of the sun directly causes cellular damage and also produces free radicals, which damage the cell walls and DNA of the skin cells.[9] If you want a graphic example of the ageing effects of the sun on your skin, compare the skin of your face to that of your underarm.

Environmental toxins

There are many other environmental toxins that contribute to the ageing process. Tobacco smoke has a profound ageing effect on the skin – not to mention on the lungs, heart and blood vessels – probably by producing free radicals. Other environmental pollutants believed to add to the free-radical load imposed on your body include:

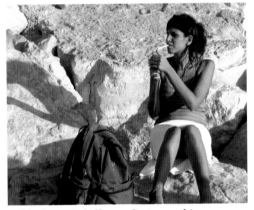

If it doesn't kill you first, smoking will certainly give you wrinkles.

❉ pesticides,

❉ X-rays,

❉ drugs,

❉ exhaust fumes.

The food we eat

The modern diet, so heavily dependent on **processed foods**, is sorely lacking in the antioxidant vitamins and minerals necessary for healthy cellular function and protection from free-radical damage. Worse, our high consumption of **refined starches**, sugars, saturated fats and animal fats actually produces free radicals and adds a significant burden of free radicals to our already nutritionally depleted body cells. An in-depth discussion of this topic is beyond the scope of this book. To read more about the nutritional aspects of ageing, see the excellent book by Dr Vincent Giampapa *et al.*[3]

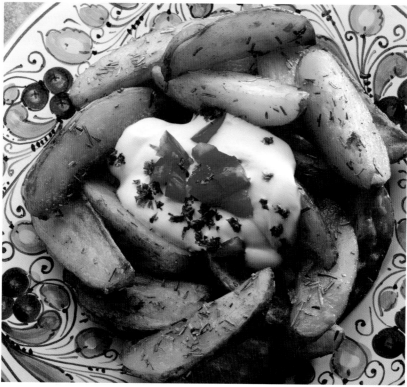

High-fat foods are a contributory factor in facial ageing.

The following are dietary products that contribute to facial ageing:

* ❦ sugar,

* ❦ alcohol,

* ❦ highly processed starches (potato crisps etc.),

* ❦ animal fats,

* ❦ barbecued and smoked meats,

* ❦ nitrate-containing or nitrite-containing foods (such as bacon),

* ❦ charred meat and fish.

Table 3.2 summarises what we have learned about the many controllable factors that contribute to the ageing process and cause the dramatic and disheartening changes we see in our faces as we age.

Table 3.2 Summary of the ageing factors

Ageing factor	Intrinsic	Extrinsic	Source	How to prevent
Cortisol modifications	X	X	Stress	Lifestyle
Dietary factors, including alcohol, refined sugars and starches, animal and saturated fats		X	Diet	Avoid
Oestrogen	X		Stress	Lifestyle modifications
Free radicals	X	X	Environment; diet; our own cells	Diet; vitamins; lifestyle modifications
Heredity	X		Genes; DNA	Human Genome Project
Human growth hormone	X		Pituitary gland	Replacement
Inflammation	X	X	Environment; diet; lifestyle	Diet; vitamins; lifestyle modifications
Melatonin	X		Pineal gland	Replacement
Progesterone	X		Ovaries	Diet; supplements; vitamins
Sunlight, ultraviolet radiation		X	Sun	Avoid sun and use sun protection
Testosterone	X		Testes	Diet; supplements; vitamins; replacement
Toxins, including X-rays, pesticides, etc.		X	Environmental; lifestyle	Avoid

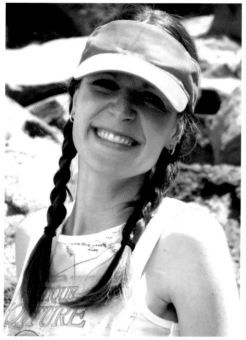

You can influence 11 of the 12 causes of facial ageing.

The good news is that of the 12 major causes of ageing, you can take definitive action to reverse or prevent 11 of them! That is very exciting news and should really motivate you to study the next chapter on prevention. Furthermore, with the exciting progress being made by the Human Genome Project, someday, in the not too distant future, we will be able to modify our genes to slow the ageing process.

Well, my cortisol levels are so high after 12 hours at the computer that my melatonin levels are getting dangerously low. I can feel the free radicals trying to initiate the inflammatory cascade in my neck and shoulders, and if I am not careful I won't be able to do any book signings. So I am going to go to sleep and let my pineal gland do its thing!

References

1. Venna, S.S. and Gilchrest, B.A. Skin ageing and photo-ageing. *Skin & Ageing* 12:56, 2004.

2. El-Domyati, M., Attia, S., Saleh, F. et al. Intrinsic ageing vs. photo-ageing: a comparative histopathological, immunohistochemical, and ultrastructural study of skin. *Exper. Dermatol.* 11:398, 2002.

3. Giampapa, V., Pero, R. and Zimmerman, M. *The Anti-aging Solution.* Hoboken, NJ: Wiley, 2004, pp. 20 and 43–5.

4. Proctor, P.H. Free radicals and human disease. *CRC Handbook of Free Radicals and Antioxidants* 1:209, 1989.

5. Meschino, J.P. *The Wrinkle Free Zone.* North Bergen, NJ: Basic Health Publications, 2004, p. 94.

6. Klatz, R. and Goldman, R. *Stopping the Clock: Longevity for the New Millennium,* 2nd edn. North Bergen, NJ: Basic Health Publications, 2002, p. 47.

7. Armstrong, S.M. and Redman, J.R. Melatonin: a chronobiotic with anti-ageing properties? *Med. Hypotheses* 34:300–9, 1991.

8. Pierpaoli, W. and Changxian, Y. The involvement of pineal gland and melatonin in immunity and ageing. *J. Neuroimmunol.* 27:99–109, 1990.

9. Nishigori, C., Hattori, Y., Arima, Y. et al. Photo-ageing and oxidative stress. *Exper. Dermatol.* 12 (Suppl. 2):18–21, 2003.

4 How to save your face – feed your mind, body and spirit

There is a major and exciting revolution in health care occurring today and you are the main beneficiary! I am talking about the anti-ageing revolution, which started many years ago. It began quietly, with a few bright, devoted scientists who knew in their hearts that Nature held the key to disease prevention and cure and longevity. Without the science to back them up, they have been viewed with suspicion by traditional medicine, and labelled as practitioners of **alternative medicine**. But science has finally caught up with the early visionaries and today we can talk seriously about effective anti-ageing strategies and start taking steps to stop and reverse the ageing of your face and your body.

Thank God for the 'alternative medicine' movement! As my father always said, 'If you want something done right, do it yourself.' This adage has never been truer than it is today with regard to your health. That is why you bought this book and that is why our generation is taking action and taking responsibility for our own health.

Fortunately, you already know about the damage free radicals can do to you and you

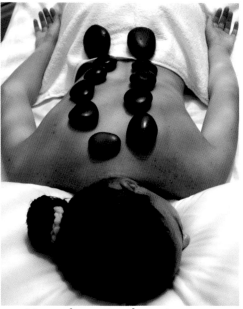

Many alternative therapies emphasise keeping yourself relaxed and healthy – prevention is better than cure.

are taking action to avoid it. It will be worth your while. Our generation is accustomed to taking the lead and not blindly accepting the status quo. Our health is the most important cause we can support.

The truth with regard to facial ageing is the same as the truth for every human disease: prevention is the best cure, or, as the saying goes, 'an ounce of prevention is worth a pound of cure'. Nowhere is that principle more evident or easier to apply than on the facial skin, our most visible and accessible body part. So let's learn what we can do to protect ourselves and prevent facial ageing.

Sun block can save your life!

Sunlight not only ages you, it can also kill you, no matter what the colour of your skin. Skin damage by the ultraviolet (UV) rays of the sun is one of the most important extrinsic causes of facial ageing. More importantly, UV light from the sun causes skin cancers: **basal cell carcinoma**, **squamous cell carcinoma** and **melanoma**. The following statistics should horrify you into taking action.

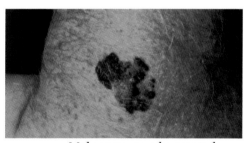

Melanoma can be treated effectively if caught early.

Invasive melanoma is a highly malignant, often fatal type of skin cancer. In 1935, Americans had a 1 in 1500 risk of developing invasive melanoma in their lifetime. This rate increased to 1 in 250 by 1980 and to 1 in 74 by 2001 and it is estimated that it will be 1 in 50 by the year 2010. Increased sun exposure, resulting from an increase in outdoor activities and more revealing clothing, as well as the increased use of tanning booths, undoubtedly play a part in this virtual epidemic. Loss of the protective ozone layer may be another important factor. A frightening fact revealed in a recent study involving teenagers in the USA is that 10 per cent use tanning booths and two-thirds don't apply sunscreens when outdoors.[1] One-third of adults in the study admitted to having suffered from sunburn in the previous year.[2] The relevant point is that sun protection is the most important yet most often neglected anti-ageing and cancer-preventing treatment you can use.

Sun block alone is not enough. New research indicates that the addition of topical antioxidant vitamins C, A and E and melatonin[3, 4, 5] significantly increases protection from the harmful effects of sunlight above and beyond the protection afforded by sun block alone. The newer sun blocks contain the antioxidant vitamins A, C, E and others.

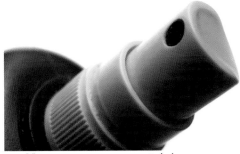

Newer sunscreens containing antioxidant vitamins are more effective.

When you are outside, exposed to the sun:

✤ Wear a wide-brimmed hat – you must protect your ears, as well as your face.

✤ Wear UV-protecting wrap-around sunglasses and sun-protective clothing, such as wet suits or 'rash guards' for children.

✤ Stay out of the sun during the peak hours, 10 a.m. to 2 p.m.

✤ Apply an even coating of sun block using 30 grams (1 ounce) for the whole body. Apply at least 30 minutes before going out in the sun.

✤ Re-apply sun block regularly every one to two hours, at minimum. Be certain to cover the area around your eyes, nose, lips and ears – the parts of your face that get the most sun, but are often missed.

✤ A sun block with SPF (sun protection factor) 15 that contains antioxidant vitamins and that blocks both UVA and UVB is a minimum. Children and adults with Type I skin (redheads) and Type II skin (fair-skinned, blue-eyed blondes) who have high sun exposure should wear a minimum of SPF 30.

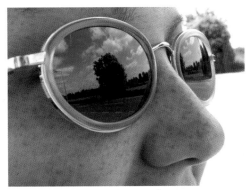

Wear UV-protecting sunglasses to protect your eyes from the sun.

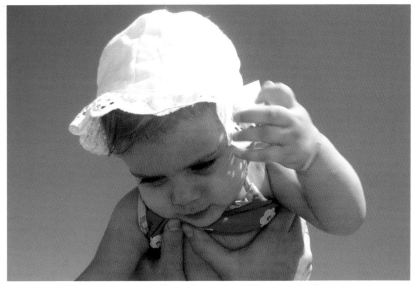

Children or those with fair skins should use a high-protection-factor sunblock.

❀ Follow the guidelines, even on cloudy days – 80 per cent of UV rays are transmitted on a cloudy day.

❀ Total protection for your children is even more important because up to 80 per cent of an individual's lifetime of sun exposure occurs during childhood.

❀ Teach your children the Australian saying SLIP, SLOP, SLAP AND WRAP – 'Slip on a shirt, slop on sunscreen, slap on a hat and wrap-around sunglasses.'

Antioxidants and nutritional supplements prevent cellular suicide

Our skin is a vibrant, living organ, the largest organ of our bodies. In Chapter 3, you learned how free-radical damage occurring in our cells causes ageing, cell death and cancer. Fortunately, Nature has provided us with natural antioxidant vitamins and minerals that work inside our cells to neutralise the damaging free radicals and make them harmless. This process is called scavenging, and the vitamins and minerals that remove free radicals are called free-radical scavengers.

It is essential that we have adequate levels of these free-radical scavengers in our cells. The way nature intended us to get these important vitamins and minerals was through our diet. Long ago, when we were 'cave men and women', we survived on the fruits, nuts and berries provided by Nature and the occasional meat we were lucky enough to obtain through hunting or scavenging the kills

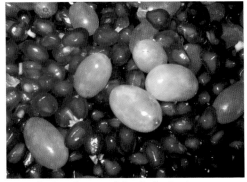

Include plenty of fresh fruits in your diet.

of larger animals, or animals that died of injury or disease. This early diet, primarily consisting of fruits and vegetables, was rich in antioxidant vitamins and minerals, complex carbohydrates and proteins, and low in fat. Obviously, this diet allowed our species to flourish and populate the Earth! In earlier times, people rarely lived long enough to develop chronic diseases such as diabetes, heart disease and arthritis; they were killed at a relatively young age – certainly before their thirties – by accident, larger animals or infections, not by old age.

As we learned to control the supply of food necessary to survive by domesticating animals and farming, our diet began to change. We learned how to process or refine starches and sugars, creating white bread from wheat and white crystallised sugar from natural sugar. We learned to domesticate and fatten livestock for a steady supply of meat with a high fat content. These developments and the

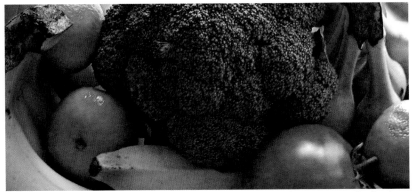

Include at least five portions of fruit and vegetables in your daily diet.

55

subsequent discovery of antibiotics to treat infections increased the human lifespan to more than 70 years. However, our new diet also set the stage for the development of many of the modern-day diseases such as diabetes, obesity, heart disease and cancer.

The processing, refining and preservation of much of our food supply remove the essential antioxidants that Nature has provided for us in the fruits and vegetables that were a dietary staple all those years ago. Worse, much of what we eat, especially fat, actually contains or creates more free radicals than the free-radical scavenger systems of our body can handle. So, you might say, what we eat is actually killing us!

As a result, it is necessary to add antioxidant vitamins and minerals and foods high in antioxidants to our diet if we want to prevent or reverse some of the free-radical-mediated damage to our facial skin. The following is a brief discussion of many of the antioxidant vitamins, minerals and compounds, and the daily dosages for supplementation of a healthy diet that are recommended by Klatz and Goldman in their book *Stopping the Clock: Longevity for the New Millennium*.[9]

Vitamin A

Vitamin A and its precursor, beta-carotene, are found in yellow, green and orange vegetables, egg yolks, liver, butter and fish oils. Vitamin A and the derivatives of vitamin A are called the **retinoids**, which are an important ingredient in many skin medications. Retinoids regulate the growth of the epidermal cells, inhibit the

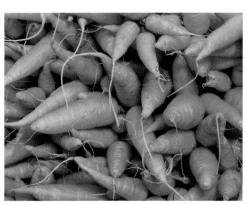

Carrots are a great source of vitamin A.

formation of cancer, decrease inflammation and improve immune function in the skin.[6, 7] Vitamin A and its derivatives are powerful antioxidants, and studies have shown that vitamin A can decrease and reverse the signs of ageing of the skin.[7] Current recommendations for supplementation are vitamin A 2500 IU/day or beta-carotene (the vitamin A precursor) 10,000 IU/day.

Vitamin A and its derivatives can cause birth defects, and excessive doses can cause increased pressure on the brain. Therefore, supplements of vitamin A and beta-carotene should not be taken by women who are pregnant and dosages higher than those recommended should be avoided.

Vitamin C

Vitamin C is a powerful antioxidant and is also important in new collagen formation, wound healing and the formation of the hormone-like **prostaglandins** PG1 and PG3, substances that play an essential role in making the skin smooth and soft. Vitamin C is also important for the regeneration of vitamin E and has been shown to enhance the skin's protection against the harmful effects of UV radiation from sunlight![7, 8] The recommended daily dosage is 1000 mg.

Vitamin E

Vitamin E is a fat-soluble vitamin, found in the cell membranes. It is an important free-radical scavenger that helps prevent damage to the cell membrane, which, you'll recall, is one of the main targets of the damage caused by free radicals. Clinically, vitamin E has been shown to have beneficial effects on **low-**

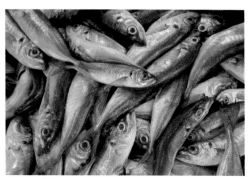

Fish is an excellent source of vitamin E.

density lipoprotein (LDL) **cholesterol**, heart disease and immune function. When too much LDL cholesterol circulates in the blood, it can slowly build up on the inner walls of the arteries that feed the heart and brain. Together with other substances, it can form plaque, a thick, hard deposit that can clog those arteries.[9] The recommended daily dose is 400 IU. The best sources of vitamin E are vegetable oils such as sunflower, canola, corn, soybean and olive oil. Nuts, sunflower seeds and wheat germ are also good sources, and vitamin E is also present in whole grains, fish, peanut butter, and green, leafy vegetables.

Vitamin E can interfere with the clotting ability of the blood, so do not take this vitamin if you are on coumadin or other blood thinners.

Selenium

Selenium is a mineral that acts as a beneficial antioxidant in cholesterol metabolism. It has been shown to have beneficial effects on heart disease, cancer and the immune system. The levels of this mineral in the body drop 7–24 per cent by the age of 70.[10] Selenium is found in Brazil nuts, sunflower seeds, grains, meat, garlic and

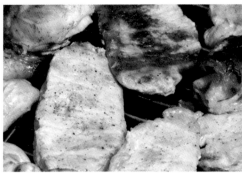

Trace elements such as selenium are found in meat.

seafood. It plays an important role in the antioxidant protection of the skin. The recommended daily dosage is 70 mcg.

Zinc

Zinc is necessary for the production of superoxide dismutase, an important antioxidant enzyme. It plays a vital role in immunity and wound healing. The recommended daily dosage is 15 mg.[11] Shellfish are high in zinc, as are liver, oxtail and corned beef. Other good

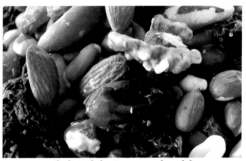

Nuts and dried fruit are a healthy snack alternative.

sources are nuts, whole grains and cheese, and zinc is also present in wheat germ, tofu, halva and figs.

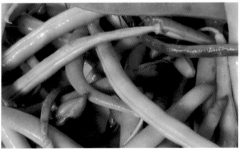

Legumes and green vegetables should be a part of your diet.

Magnesium

Magnesium participates in antioxidant activity that protects cell membranes and the mitochondria, and is also very important in regulating calcium balance. It is found in whole grains, nuts, seeds and legumes. The recommended daily dose is 400 mg.[12]

Coenzyme Q10

Coenzyme Q10 is necessary for the production of enzyme Q10 in the mitochondria in cells. It also acts as an antioxidant, protecting the cell membrane.[13] Recently, coenzyme Q10 has been used to reverse congestive heart failure,[14] although there have also been controlled clinical studies that have failed to show any beneficial effect in this role.[15]

The **statin drugs** used to lower cholesterol can deplete coenzyme Q10.[16] The recommended daily dose of coenzyme Q10 is 30–280 mg. Coenzyme Q10 is sold as a nutritional supplement and therefore there are no established dosage guidelines. Adults typically use a coenzyme Q10 supplement that provides between 30 mg and 100 mg per day, although people with specific health conditions may supplement with higher levels (with the involvement of a physician). Most of the clinical studies conducted on heart conditions have used 60–150 mg of coenzyme Q10 per day. However, coenzyme Q10 can interact with many other drugs, so you should consult your doctor before taking it.

Alpha-lipoic acid

Alpha-lipoic acid (ALA) is important in the regeneration of the antioxidants vitamin C, vitamin E and coenzyme Q10, and helps protect DNA from metals that can generate free radicals.[17] ALA can also help prevent **glycation**, which has a harmful effect on the sugar in the blood. The recommended daily dose is 100 mg.[18]

L-Carnitine

L-Carnitine assists in the transport of fats across the cell membrane and thus in the burning of fats for energy production. It is also important in enhancing the effects of coenzyme Q10. The recommended daily dose is 50–100 mg per day.[19]

Sulphur-containing antioxidants

Sulphur-containing vegetables such as **cruciferous vegetables** (e.g. cauliflower and broccoli) and garlic have antioxidant properties and are important for immune function. The recommended daily dosage is extract of cruciferous vegetables 500–1000 mg, and garlic 100 mg.[20]

Repair your DNA – carboxy alkyl esters

In Chapter 3, we discussed the crucial role of DNA damage in the ageing process. There is exciting new evidence that it may be possible to reverse DNA damage. Dr Ron Pero, a molecular biologist in Lund, Sweden, has isolated a group of compounds called carboxy alkyl esters (CAEs), which he purports actually stimulate DNA repair enzymes when paired with nicotinamide (a B vitamin), zinc and natural carotenes. The author cites studies that show that these compounds can improve immunity and decrease inflammation. He recommends a daily dose of CAE extract of 350 mg taken with medicinal mushroom extracts 500–1000 mg.[21]

Fatty acid supplements

Whereas most animal fats are harmful, the fatty acids known as omega-3 oils have many positive health benefits. Remember how the cell wall contains fats and that fats play an essential role in protecting your skin? Cold-water fish and dark-green vegetables are natural sources of good fatty acids. Dr Giampapa[22] recommends a fish omega-3 blend of eicosapentaenoic acid (EPA) 300 mg and docosahexaenoic acid (DHA) 200 mg, three capsules per day for cardiovascular and immune benefits.

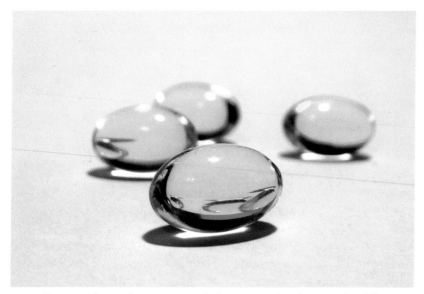

Fatty-acid supplements can help you maintain your health.

B vitamins

The B vitamins play an important role in skin health. Deficiency syndromes include cracks in the lips (B2 [riboflavin] deficiency), pellagra (a condition causing a rash and rough skin due to B3 [niacin] deficiency) and skin pigmentation (vitamin B12 deficiency). Vitamin B5, also known as panthenol, the active form of panthothenic acid, is widely used as a humectant (moisturiser) for the skin. Vitamin B3 and B6 also play a role in the synthesis of prostaglandin, which helps maintain skin softness. The B vitamins are important in cellular energy production, the protection of DNA and the proper function of the genes. Taking a B-50 complex vitamin daily is recommended for optimal skin health.[23] Vitamin B comes from a number of natural sources, including potatoes, bananas, lentils, chilli peppers, tempeh, liver, turkey, tuna and brewers' yeast.

Prostaglandins

The hormone-like prostaglandins are made by skin cells from fats in the diet. PG1 and PG3 work together to moisten the skin and make it soft. They are not to be confused with PG2, which is a harmful by-product of the oxidation product arachidonic acid. According to Dr Meschino,[24] PG1 synthesis is optimised by supplementation with borage oil, and PG3 synthesis is enhanced by supplementing with fish oil and flaxseed oil. He recommends the following.

* Reduce your intake of high-fat meats and dairy products, which increase PG2 synthesis.

* Substitute olive oil, canola oil and/or peanut oil in place of corn, sunflower, safflower seed and mixed vegetable oils.

Detoxification – remove skin-damaging toxins from your body

The liver is the primary organ in the body responsible for **detoxification** – that is, making harmless, dangerous substances that have accumulated in the blood. The liver detoxifies the excess hormones and other chemicals produced by our bodies, as well as medications, alcohol, pesticides and other environmental contaminants. As we age, our liver detoxification system can slow down due to the accumulation of toxic substances or as the result of damage by alcohol, age or diseases such as hepatitis. Failure of liver detoxification can allow harmful toxic substances to build up in the blood, many of which are free radicals and can increase skin-ageing changes. Dr Meschino[25] recommends a daily detoxification protocol for optimum skin health and anti-ageing nutritional support. His recommendations are listed in the protocol below.

Detoxification protocol

* Cruciferous vegetables (e.g. broccoli).

* Grapefruit, oranges.

* Soy extract.

* Milk thistle 150–600 mg.

* Vitamin C 1000 mg.

* Indole-3 carbinol 25–100 mg.

* Reischi mushroom extract 30–120 mg.

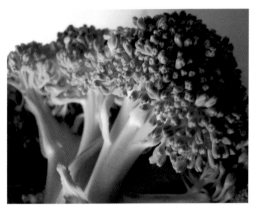

Cruciferous vegetables such as broccoli are one of the superfoods.

* Astragalus 100–400 mg.

* Low-fat yoghurt.

* Fermented foods (yoghurt).

Detoxification is inhibited by:

* antidepressants

* antihistamines

* bacterial toxins

* ageing.

Digestive enzyme deficiency and intestinal dysbiosis

The proper digestion of food requires the presence of various enzymes within the digestive tract to break down the food we eat into appropriately sized protein molecules. These protein molecules can then be taken up by the cells of the digestive tract, passed into the bloodstream and carried to individual cells where the proteins are metabolised.

Insufficient digestion of food, caused by a lack of the appropriate enzymes in the intestine, can lead to improperly or partially digested food proteins entering the bloodstream. These improperly digested foreign proteins can initiate an autoimmune or immune inflammatory reaction, whereby we make antibodies that attack our own bodies. This digestive enzyme deficiency is also called **intestinal dysbiosis**, and can aggravate many skin conditions such as **psoriasis, rosacea, acne** and **eczema**.

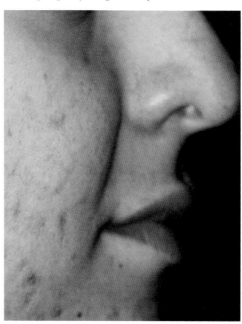

Acne can be a response to a digestive disorder.

In addition, frequent use of powerful antibiotics – which are used to treat infections and are present in our food supply – combined with high-fat, low-fibre diets can result in damage to the 'friendly' bacteria that are normally present in the large intestine (colon). In some cases, the useful bacteria in the gut become too abundant and produce toxins, which then enter the bloodstream and cause an immune, inflammatory reaction that can damage the skin.

How do we restore balance to the intestinal flora? By decreasing fat in the diet, by increasing our intake of fibre and yoghurt and other fermented foods high in *Lactobacillus* bacteria, and by the detoxification regimen listed above, as suggested by Dr Meschino.

Women's hormonal balance

Pre-menopausal

The female sex hormones oestrogen and progesterone, discussed in Chapter 3, have important effects on the skin. High oestrogen-to-progesterone ratios are associated with pre-menstrual syndrome (PMS), fibrocystic breast disease, uterine fibroids and endometriosis. Table 4.1 shows the factors that can aggravate and improve a high oestrogen:progestin ratio.[26]

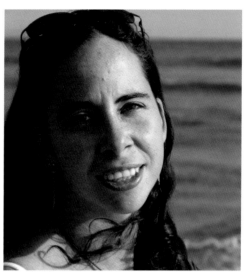

Female hormone levels also have an impact on your skin.

Table 4.1 Factors that can cause or improve a high oestrogen:progesterone ratio

Causes of high oestrogen: progesterone	Factors that improve oestrogen: progesterone balance
High-fat diet	Low-fat, higher-fibre diet
Low fibre intake	Aerobic exercise
Intestinal dysbiosis	Correct intestinal dysbiosis
Poor liver detoxification	Improve detoxification
Corpus luteum failure (ovarian failure)	Black cohosh
	Soy isoflavones
	Gamma-oryzanol

Peri-menopausal and post-menopausal

As discussed in Chapter 3, menopause brings a 90 per cent decline in oestrogen levels and a 66 per cent decline in progesterone levels. These hormonal declines cause many of the symptoms of menopause, including the well-known ones – hot flashes, sweats, insomnia, anxiety and irritability.

Whereas oestrogen therapy or hormone replacement therapy (HRT) can abate the symptoms associated with menopause, there are risks associated with the latter. HRT has been shown to be associated with an increase in the risk of breast cancer, heart attack, stroke and possibly ovarian cancer. Furthermore, in pre-menopausal women who have had breast cancer, oestrogen suppression therapy with drugs such as tamoxifen can also result in menopausal symptoms that have a profound ageing effect on the skin of these younger women.

The following holistic or alternative therapies have been successful in Europe and Asia and do not have the risks of HRT.[27]

* ❧ Black cohosh 160 mg per day.

* ❧ Soy isoflavones 50–75 mg per day.

* ❧ Gamma-oryzanol 300 mg per day.

Other important anti-ageing hormones

Hormones are complex, highly biologically active substances, and hormone supplements should only be used under the direction of a physician, preferably an **endocrinologist**. The unfortunate lesson we learned from HRT and oestrogen therapy is that hormones can stimulate the growth of cancer. Therefore hormone supplements should be used only when you have a documented deficiency that has been determined by tests to assess the levels of hormones in your blood. The following discussion is for informational purposes and is not a recommendation that you take these substances without a doctor's prescription.

Dehydroepiandrosterone

Dehydroepiandrosterone (DHEA) is a steroid hormone, the most abundant hormone in the body, and is involved in the production of many other hormones, including progesterone, oestrogen and testosterone.

The literature suggests that DHEA levels fall with ageing and their restoration can result

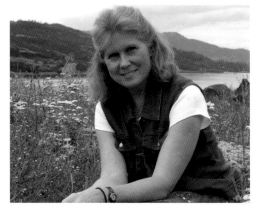

There are better alternatives to HRT for menopausal women.

in improved immune function, the restoration of lean muscle mass and improvement in the many bodily functions that decline with age. The problem is that if you take this hormone when you are not deficient, bad things can happen.

Have you heard of the muscular body builders who have atrophied testicles and cannot produce sperm? Abuse of DHEA is the culprit. A doctor friend of mine once told me he was taking DHEA for its anti-ageing properties and he was kind enough to send me a bottle. Several months later, he told me he had developed prostate cancer! Coincidence, you say? Maybe, but the pills went into the trash. The US Food and Drug Administration (FDA) is trying hard to control the abuse of this powerful and too readily available hormone supplement.

Human growth hormone

Human growth hormone (hGH) has dramatic age-reversing effects, especially when given to people who are deficient in this hormone. Improvements in the skin, lean body muscle mass, energy, libido and general well-being are reported. However, as pointed out in Chapter 3, hGH stimulates cell division – and cancer is unregulated cell division. Doctor Andy Guay, a respected endocrinologist at Lahey Clinic in Boston, USA, fears that taking hGH when you do not have a documented deficiency could 'turn on' cells predisposed to cancer. If you might be interested in taking hGH, see an endocrinologist and have your blood levels tested.

However, according to expert medical opinion, oral hGH preparations do not work. For hGH to be effective, you need to take daily injections, which is a good thing because it discourages most people. Don't be ripped off by those Internet 'pop ups' that promise you the fountain of youth by taking hGH in pill or spray form. Taking hGH pills is like putting aspirin on the top of your head for a headache!

Thyroid hormone

If you are deficient in **thyroid hormone**, you are hypothyroid and must be under the care of an endocrinologist. If you are clinically deficient, thyroid hormone will improve your bodily functions. If you are not deficient, thyroid hormone can hurt you, so don't take it!

Melatonin

As discussed in Chapter 3, melatonin (which is produced by the pineal gland) is an important antioxidant that has specific protective effects on the immune system to prevent inflammation. Stress reduces our melatonin levels. Melatonin is readily available in tablet form, and widely used as a sleep aid and to prevent 'jet lag'. Studies have shown that melatonin supplementation with 0.5–5 mg is safe.[9] Transdermal patches are also available.

Food – you are what you eat

It is obvious that our diet plays a profound role in our overall health and in the ageing process. There are excellent books on healthy eating and painstakingly detailed descriptions of wholesome anti-ageing diets full of antioxidants and other important elements.[18, 19] These are useful sources for detailed menu plans.

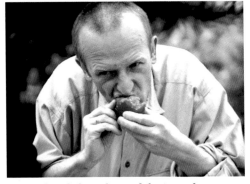

Eat brightly coloured fruit and vegetables as part of your healthy diet.

The following are general dietary but critical guidelines for you to follow if you are serious about preventing – and possibly reversing – ageing changes to your facial skin.

- ✿ Eat more fish, especially cold-water fish such as salmon.

- ✿ Eat more brightly coloured and cruciferous vegetables.

- ✿ Eat more fibre.

- ✿ Eat more soy products.

- ✿ Eat fewer animal and hydrogenated fats.

- ✿ Eat less refined sugar.

- ✿ Drink less alcohol.

I am aware that some authors today are advocating 'eat, drink and be merry'. If you are thin, healthy and active and have a genetic profile compatible with longevity, then you are blessed and may survive ignoring important dietary principles. For the rest of us mere mortals, dietary modification is an essential component for healthy longevity.

Avoid sources high in free radicals. Known sources of free radicals[28] are:

❀ UV light from the sun,

❀ cigarette smoke,

❀ alcohol,

❀ smoked or barbequed foods,

❀ nitrosamines (bacon and other preserved foods),

❀ heavy metals – lead etc.,

❀ X-rays,

❀ sugar,

❀ pesticides.

Nutritional anti-ageing checklist for your skin and face (a cheat sheet)

For all skin types

❀ Reduce your intake of high-animal-fat products (meat and dairy), which lower arachidonic acid (AA) levels.

❀ Reduce your intake of vegetable oils, which include corn, safflower seed and mixed vegetable oils, which lower **linoleic acid** (LA) – high amounts of LA convert to AA.

❀ Restrict your alcohol intake.

❀ Reduce your intake of hydrogenated fats.

❀ Reduce your intake of refined sugars.

❀ Do not smoke.

❀ Increase your intake of cruciferous vegetables, which include broccoli, cauliflower and cabbage.

❀ Increase your intake of soy-based products.

❦ Increase your intake of protein by having a soy-based – or whey-based – protein shake daily.

❦ Drink ten glasses of water daily.

❦ Increase your intake of fruits high in vitamin C – oranges are an excellent choice.

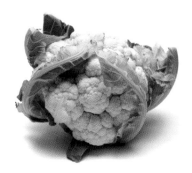

Cauliflower is on the list of positive foods for all skin types.

❦ Increase your intake of vegetables – the more colourful, the better.

❦ Increase your intake of fish – wild salmon is an excellent choice and is high in omega-3 oil.

❦ Wear sunscreen with an SPF of at least 15 and re-apply it throughout the day if you are outdoors.

Recommended daily doses of antioxidants

❦ Vitamin C 1000 mg.

❦ Vitamin E 400 IU.

❦ Beta-carotene 10,000 IU.

❦ Selenium 70 mcg.

❦ Zinc 15 mg.

❦ Lycopene 6 mg.

❦ Lutein 6 mg.

Daily detox plan

❦ Cruciferous vegetables.

❦ Oranges (contain limonene, which is a flavonoid).

❦ Soy isoflavones.

❦ Soy extract (supplement in a protein shake).

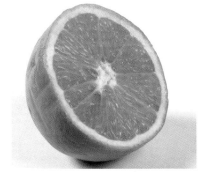

Oranges are a source of vitamin C and the flavonoid limonene.

- ❦ Milk thistle (a powerful detoxifier) 150–600 mg.

- ❦ Vitamin C 1000 mg.

- ❦ Indole-3-carbinol 25–100 mg.

- ❦ Reishi mushroom extract 30–120 mg.

- ❦ Astragalus 100–400 mg.

- ❦ Low-fat yoghurt and other fermented foods that deliver good bacteria.

- ❦ Fibre. For women younger than 50, 25 g per day, and for those older than 50, 21 g per day. For men younger than 50, 38 g per day, and for those older than 50, 30 g per day.

Women's hormonal balance

- ❦ Black cohosh 160 mg.

- ❦ Soy extract 500 mg.

- ❦ Gamma-oryzanol 300 mg.

Men's prostate balance

- ❦ Saw palmetto 320 mg twice a day.

- ❦ Pygeum Africanum 100 mg twice a day.

- ❦ Beta-sitosterol 65 mg twice a day.

- ❦ Soy extract 200 mg twice a day.

- ❦ Stinging nettle 30 mg twice a day.

- ❦ Lycopene extract 12.5 mg a day.

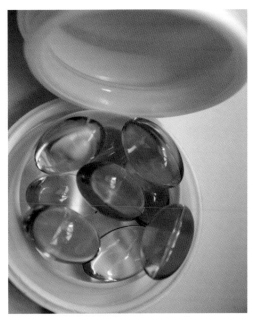

Choose your supplements wisely to improve your intake of nutrients.

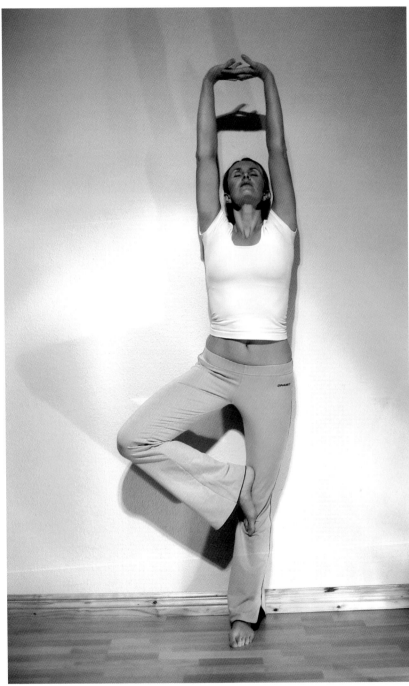

Exercise such as yoga has major health and well-being benefits.

Change your lifestyle

Modification of your lifestyle is one of the most important and effective steps you can take to improve your overall health and prevent ageing. Avoiding alcohol, tobacco and 'recreational drugs' is essential for good health. Want proof? Look into the face of someone who abuses these things and you will be immediately convinced of the terrible effects of these toxins on the beauty and vitality of the human face.

Stress and the sedentary lifestyle – our most self-destructive behaviours

Stress

Stress is a major factor in many modern diseases, including ageing. Chronic stress elevates the levels of cortisol in the body and, as we learned in Chapter 3, cortisol is referred to as the age-accelerating hormone. Dr Giampapa writes that the primary source of stress in our lives is **time urgency**, the feeling we get when we set ourselves up to accomplish three or four tasks when we have the time to do just one.[19]

In addition, especially for those of us who live or work in large metropolitan areas, crowding, noise, crime and a steady diet of anxiety-provoking news make it nearly impossible to maintain a peaceful state of mind. Many people are finding that meditation and yoga are helpful antidotes for stress, a notion that is supported by some scientific medical studies.[29]

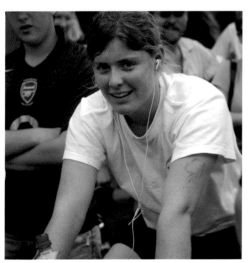

Choose an exercise you enjoy and make it part of your routine.

Exercise

Exercise is essential for good health and is one of the most effective anti-ageing strategies. However, some intriguing new research suggests that intensive 'weekend warrior' exercise is counterproductive to good health. More moderate forms of exercise, such as resistance weight training, moderate aerobic exercise, walking and yoga, are better for our bodies and have more meaningful health-promoting and longevity-promoting benefits. There are hundreds of books on exercise, but Dr Giampapa's exercise programme is specifically geared towards anti-ageing and is backed by sound scientific evidence.[19]

The following are the most important points about exercise.

- Choose something you enjoy – that way you'll be able to maintain your enthusiasm.

- Commitment: decide that you are going to incorporate some form of exercise into each day.

- Stretch before and after you exercise.

- Resistance: include some weight training in your routine; repetitions are more important than the amount of weight.

- Aerobic exercise: important for your heart and to release endorphins, which improve your mood. Include a 30-minute period in which your heart rate increases to the safe level for your age and health status.

- Yoga: the health benefits of yoga are becoming widely recognised and many gyms now offer programmes.

Spirituality – the key to healthy longevity and a radiant face

For me, it is easier to define spirituality by stating what it is not. Many define the whole person as consisting of the body, mind and spirit. Spirituality is something we experience that is not in the realm of the body or the mind. It is a profoundly personal experience. Religion in any form is one way in which

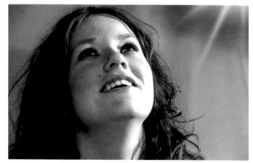

Spirituality has an elevating effect on the spirit.

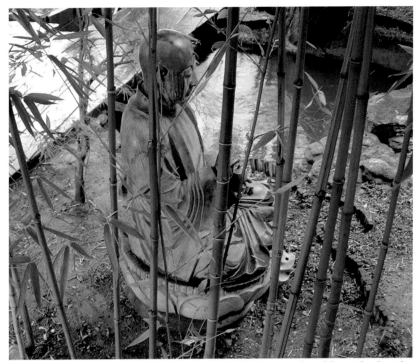

People with a spiritual component to their lives may be able to deal with stress more effectively.

many people understand or express their personal concept of spirit, but although all people have a spiritual component to their being, not all people are religious.

The reason I include a discussion of spirituality here is because I believe, based on my 30 years of experience as a doctor, that spiritually connected people handle most forms of stress more effectively – as we know, stress is a major factor in accelerating the ageing of the skin and body. The importance of spirituality in promoting good health and recovery from illness or injury is increasingly being recognised by the contemporary medical community.[30]

A recent study showed that a large number of members of the younger generation of college students place high importance on spirituality. In a survey of third-year college students in the USA, 58 per cent felt that integrating spirituality in life is very important or essential; 77 per cent of those who responded said that they pray; 73 per cent said their spiritual/religious beliefs helped them develop

their identity.[31] In addition, millions of people worldwide have been released from the burden of addiction to drugs, food, alcohol and other destructive behaviours by
12-step programmes, which are all based on spirituality and belief in a higher power.

No one can explain why, but spirituality elevates us. I know a spiritual person when I meet one. I'm sure you do too. To me, spirituality requires humility and the acknowledgement that, no matter what our abilities are, there is a higher power, force, consciousness or whatever you want to call it that is overwhelmingly benign. If we acknowledge it, we will be released from the burden of self-will. Failure to acknowledge a force greater than ourselves leaves us with the horrendous burden of being responsible for many things over which we really have no control. That burden, in my opinion, creates stress, anxiety and worry – all of which are not only reflected on our faces by frown lines and worry lines, but also negatively impact our entire body.

I am referring to **coronary artery disease**, heart attacks, high blood pressure, stroke, mental illness, addictions and who knows how many more stress-related diseases. So I strongly urge you to incorporate your own spiritual programme into your daily life. There are so many to choose from – organised Western religions, Buddhism, you name it. For some, it may mean communing with nature or simply enjoying a beautiful painting. For me, the essential ingredient is a belief in some higher power that is responsible for our existence and experience. Armed with this humility, we can be open to experience the wonderful opportunities that are presented to us. Freed from the bonds of self-will, we will be less stressed and happier and our faces will show it. We will age less harshly and certainly in a less stressful and more healthful way.

Isn't it fascinating that we have been given the miracle of **Botox**™ to erase frown lines and worry lines, but we cannot use this drug to reduce smile lines, because to do so would deform the face. There is a message in there for those willing to listen!

References
1. Lim, H.W., Naylor, M., Honigsmann, H. et al. American Academy of Dermatology Consensus Conference on UVA Protection of Sunscreens: summary and recommendations. *J. Am. Acad. Dermatol.* 44:505, 2001.
2. DiGironimo, G. Skin cancer update: sunning yourself to death. *Skin & Ageing* 10:16, 2002.
3. Tuleya, S. Skin cancer and photo-ageing update. *Skin & Ageing* 11:40, 2003.

4. Pinnell, S.R. Cutaneous photo-damage, oxidative stress, and topical antioxidant protection. *J. Am. Acad. Dermatol.* 48:1, 2003.

5. Fischer, T. and Elsner, E. The antioxidative potential of melatonin in the skin. In Thiele, J. and Elsner, P. (eds), *Oxidants and antioxidants in cutaneous biology*. Current Problems in Dermatology, Vol. 29. Basil: Karger, 2001, pp. 165–74.

6. Draelos, Z.D. Evaluating vitamin formulations. *J. Aesthetic Dermatol. Cos. Surg.* 1:121, 1999.

7. Del Rosso, J.Q. Topical retinoid therapy. *Skin & Ageing* 10:50, 2002.

8. Fitzpatrick, R.E. and Rostan, E.F. Double-blind, half-face study comparing topical vitamin C and vehicle for rejuvenation of photo-damage. *Dermatol. Surg.* 28:231, 2002.

9. Klatz, R. and Goldman, R. *Stopping the Clock: Longevity for the New Millennium*, 2nd edn. North Bergen, NJ: Basic Health Publications, 2002. pp. 188–92.

10. As above, pp. 163–7.

11. As above, pp. 216–19.

12. As above, pp. 167–72.

13. As above, pp. 198–202.

14. Khatta, M., Alexander, B.S., Krichten, C.M. et al. The effect of coenzyme Q10 in patients with congestive heart failure. *Ann. Intern. Med.* 132:636, 2000.

15. Watson, P.S., Scalia, G.M., Galbraith, A. et al. Lack of effect of coenzyme Q on left ventricular function in patients with congestive heart failure. J. Am. Coll. Cardiol. 33:1549, 1999.

16. Bliznakov, E.G. Coenzyme Q10 lipid-lowering drugs (statins) and cholesterol: a present day Pandora's Box. *J. A. N. A.* 5:32, 2002.

17. Packer, L., Witt, E.H., Tritschler, H.J. Alpha-lipoic acid as a biological antioxidant. *Free Rad. Biol. Med.* 19:227, 1995.

18. Perricone, N. *The Perricone Prescription*, 1st edn. New York: Harper Collins, 2002, p. 78.

19. Giampapa, V., Pero, R. and Zimmerman, M. *The Anti-aging Solution*. Hoboken, NJ: Wiley, 2004, p. 138.

20. As above, p. 136.

21. As above, pp. 141–4.

22. As above, pp. 147–8.

23. Meschino, J.P. *The Wrinkle Free Zone*. North Bergen, NJ: Basic Health Publications, 2004, p. 41.

24. As above, p. 23.

25. As above, p. 58.

26. As above, p. 94.

27. As above, p. 134.

28. As above, pp. 25–30.

29. Vyas, R. and Dikshit, N. Effect of meditation on respiratory system, cardiovascular system, and lipid profile. *Indian J. Physiol. Pharmacol.* 46:487, 2002.

30. Dossy, L. Prayer and medical science. *Arch. Int. Med.* 160:1735, 2000.

31. College students express strong interest in spirituality and high levels of tolerance for religious diversity and the non-religious. *AAC & U News* Feb. 2004.

5 Dr Seckel's 6-Step Non-Surgical Facial Rejuvenation Program®

In Chapter 4 I wrote that 'There is a major and exciting revolution in health care occurring today and you are the main beneficiary.' Nowhere in the field of anti-ageing medicine are the breakthroughs and technological advances more exciting, more relevant and more readily available for immediate application and benefit to you than in the field of facial rejuvenation. Better, the most exciting, *effective* new discoveries are *non-surgical* methods for facial rejuvenation. Yes, I said 'non-surgical' and I said 'effective'.

Today's breakthrough therapies are effective – you will see a younger face staring back at you in the mirror. The six-step programme described below produces results that you can actually see! No prolonged, complicated diets, no magical creams, no miracle cure that insults your intelligence, takes your money and after 6 months to a year changes nothing in your appearance, leaving you too dispirited or disgusted to ask for your money back.

I have been a **plastic surgeon** for over 23 years and can perform surgical procedures that restore a face to a youthful appearance in a very short time, but my experience has taught me that no one wants to have surgery – there

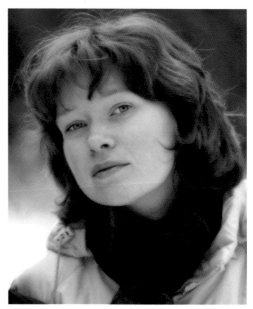

My 6-step programme can help you maintain your youthful looks.

must be a better way. I became aware, beginning with the advances in laser therapy in 1995, that non-surgical facial rejuvenation was possible, yet the technology needed further development for effective non-surgical rejuvenation to become a reality. Several new scientific advances were made during the past 3 years that have made non-surgical rejuvenation truly possible for many of you today.

I have developed a non-surgical programme consisting of six basic steps, each step designed to correct a specific facial ageing change. When these steps are used in the correct sequence on the face of a properly selected individual, true rejuvenation to a more youthful-looking face is possible. Dry skin, wrinkles, brown spots, blood vessels and, for some, even loose skin are all improved.

I know you are anxious to get to the heart of this subject and my six-step programme, but I want you first to understand what makes the face look old. Only then will you be able to evaluate your own face and seek the appropriate therapies outlined in the programme. So please read the section below. How do we change from that radiant 16-year-old with smooth, glowing, fresh skin to a 40-something who is beginning to see her mother looking back at her in the mirror, to a 65-year-old with hooded eyes, puffy lower eyelids, jowls and loose skin folds hanging under the chin?

This transformation is a clearly understood physiological process called ageing and is accelerated by sun damage and inflammation. But if you think sun block, creams and diet will correct these changes once you have them, you have a very sad and disappointing surprise awaiting you in the years ahead. While prevention is very important – most important to prevent skin cancer – the visible ageing changes that make you look old and tired are structural, anatomic, genetically determined changes in your skin that are going to occur to some degree no matter how well you take care of yourself. You need outside help; you will need to take action if you want to keep a youthful facial appearance. The appropriate actions, which lead to effective correction of these changes, are clearly outlined in my six-step programme, which follows. But first let's review what we learned in Chapters 1 and 2 and make sure we clearly understand what changes we must look for, recognise and then take steps to correct.

Let's consider the characteristics of the woman's face on the following page that make her look older than the child.

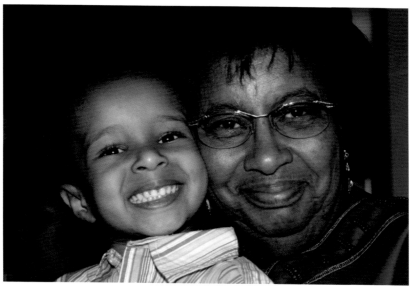

It is easy to see how age changes our facial appearance.

❧ *Skin texture changes.* The woman's facial skin looks dry when compared with the child's skin. Over half of the crucial natural skin-moisturising agent hyaluronic acid is lost by the time we turn 50. You cannot replace hyaluronic acid by taking a pill or applying it to your skin. Loss of hormonal support during menopause accelerates this change. Dry, aged skin loses its glow and looks dull. The aged skin is also wrinkled and rough and pore size is enlarged. Sometimes there are dry, flaking patches of skin on the surface of the face.

❧ *Uneven pigmentation, brown spots, red spots and blood vessels.* Uneven pigmentation and overgrowth of blood vessels are characteristic of aged facial skin. These blemishes are the skin's protective and inflammatory response to years of exposure to ultraviolet (UV) light from the sun and injury from free radicals released by harmful agents in our environment and diet.

❧ *Fine lines and wrinkles.* Fine lines and wrinkles are classic signs of facial ageing. **Static wrinkles** are those that are present in the skin when the face is at rest. These are caused by the loss of collagen in the deeper layers of the skin. Collagen is destroyed by UV light from the sun and by free radicals from other sources. As the collagen disappears, volume is lost beneath the skin and the skin wrinkles. This is not unlike the way a grape wrinkles after drying to produce a raisin. **Dynamic wrinkles** are those that you see when the face is moving – frown lines, laugh lines, worry lines and crow's feet. These lines are actually caused by the pull of the facial muscles beneath the skin. Dynamic wrinkles can become static wrinkles after years of repeated pulling by the facial muscles.

✤ *Deep facial lines.* Deep facial lines are the lines around the mouth, the nasal–labial fold line and the marionette lines. These lines are different from wrinkles in that they are caused by a combination of the pull of the facial muscles and loose, sagging skin. As the face ages, the skin becomes loose and falls over the line created by the facial muscle pull, for example the smile line.

✤ *Loose skin.* The skin of an older person's face loses its elasticity and becomes loose. The cheek has fallen and created loose skin on the jaw, called jowls. The skin beneath the jaw on the neck is also hanging down, a phenomenon called the turkey wattle.

What is facial rejuvenation?

To rejuvenate is to make young or youthful again or to restore to an original or new state. True facial rejuvenation – for the face to be made young or youthful or restored to an original state – requires correction of all the facial ageing changes mentioned above. The problem with most of the wrinkle cures and anti-ageing therapies available today is that they address only one or two of the five major facial ageing changes discussed above. Treating one or two of the ageing changes is a partial treatment and achieves only a partial result, not true facial rejuvenation. For example, a **face-lift** tightens the facial skin, but you simply have tightened, old-looking skin when you are finished – better, but still old looking. Some laser procedures can remove brown spots and blood vessels and refresh the skin, but the wrinkles and sagging skin remain unchanged and the face still looks old. Botox™ can remove frown lines and crow's feet, but it does nothing about pigment, blood vessels, loose skin and other wrinkles. **Fillers** like Restylane™, Sculptra™ and Radiesse™ can soften deep lines around the mouth and nose, but do not address any of the other changes.

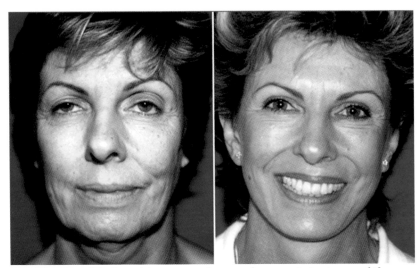

The face-lift that this woman has undergone is just one of the different procedures that can be done to improve different aspects of facial ageing.

Wrinkle creams and fad diets achieve the most disappointing results. All would agree that sun block, a healthy diet, drinking lots of water, and antioxidant vitamins are important for your health. If started when you are 16 or 18 years old, these preventative therapies may help prevent facial ageing. But once you have the physical signs of ageing, more aggressive therapy is required to reverse them and rejuvenate the face.

The good news is that we now have effective non-surgical therapies that can reverse many of the facial ageing changes. The problem is that these therapies must be applied in a step-by-step, coherent manner for truly effective rejuvenation. Too often the new facial rejuvenation therapies are

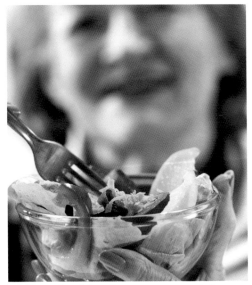

A healthy diet is an essential component of good health.

applied in a hit-or-miss fashion, with disappointing results. Many doctors, even those who specialise in facial aesthetics, are 'married to one therapy' – that is, they use a technique they understand and believe in but do not appreciate that an aged facial appearance is caused by several factors, not one or two. The fact that he or she is trained in only one or two modalities – say Botox" and fillers – may limit the doctor, who may be able to correct your crow's feet and soften the lines around your mouth and nose, but will be able to do nothing for the pigment, vessels, static wrinkles and loose skin that make your face look tired and old. Another doctor may be a laser specialist and address pigment and vessels but fail at skin tightening. Another doctor may offer you only surgery.

I call this the 'when your only tool is a hammer the whole world looks like a nail' approach. The doctors try to fit your unique face into their systematic therapy. For effective facial rejuvenation, it must be the other way around: the therapy must be adjusted and modified to fit your unique face. With the six-step programme, you get what you need for true facial rejuvenation – all major facial ageing changes are addressed, not one or two.

The 6-Step Non-surgical Facial Rejuvenation Program®

The 6-Step Non-surgical Facial Rejuvenation Program® consists of the following six steps.

1. Exfoliation.

2. Stimulation of new collagen formation.

3. Removal of abnormal pigment and blood vessels.

4. Relaxation of the muscles of facial expression.

5. Filling of deep facial lines.

6. Skin tightening.

These six steps address the major facial ageing changes that many people begin to see sometime between the ages of 30 and 50, and which are present in the faces of most people between the ages of 50 and 60. Many of you may not have all the classic facial ageing changes, and for you, the six-step programme can be customised for your unique face. However, the six-step programme is designed to address all the important facial ageing changes. Although individual steps can be done without the others for people who have only one or two changes, most people need to be on a programme that addresses all six ageing changes on an ongoing basis. Each step is discussed in detail below.

Step 1: Exfoliation

Exfoliation involves the mechanical or chemical removal of dead skin cells from the surface of the face. It contributes several beneficial rejuvenating effects to the skin surface.

1. Removal of dead skin cells: the outer surface of the skin has many layers of dead skin cells that have been pushed upwards to the skin surface by the actively growing new skin cells in the deep basal cell layer of the epidermis. These new cells are plumper and have more moisture and after the dead cells are removed by exfoliation, they are exposed and reveal a healthy, glowing and more youthful cast to the skin surface.

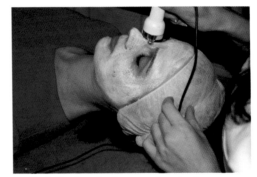

Exfoliation is the mechanical removal of dead skin cells.

2. Better penetration of rejuvenating **topical agents**: the dead skin cells form a barrier to the penetration of topically applied agents intended to remove pigmentation and stimulate new skin cell formation in the epidermis and collagen production in the dermis.

3. Removal of skin-pore-blocking debris: dead skin cells, dirt, environmental debris and skin oils accumulate on the surface of the skin and block the pores. This blockage can lead to accumulation of skin oils and sweat, which can cause milia (small cysts) and acne and result in an uneven texture to the skin and enlarged pores.

4. Mild irritation of the dermis: stronger exfoliants such as glycolic acid, **Retin-A**™, and microdermabrasion can produce mild dermal irritation and actually result in the formation of new collagen deposition in the superficial dermis.

5. Removal of superficial epidermal pigmentation: superficial pigmentation (brown spots) is a classic Type I facial ageing change. Much of this pigmentation, which is present in the epidermis, can be removed with vigorous exfoliation, which also allows topical agents intended to remove pigment in the deeper layers to penetrate the skin more easily to exert their effect.

Step 2: Stimulation of new collagen formation

Since the major factor contributing to the ageing of the facial skin is damage to, and loss of, the dermal collagen, an important component of any facial rejuvenation programme is the stimulation of new collagen production in the dermis. Producing new collagen in the dermis of the skin has several major benefits.

1. It increases dermal thickness and counteracts the thinning that characterises ageing facial skin.

2. It has a plumping or filling effect on the age-damaged areas of the dermis that have atrophied and resulted in the depressions that underlie wrinkles. This plumping effect can reduce the depth and number of facial wrinkles.

3. It can more effectively provide nutritional support for the overlying epidermis and result in a healthier, fresher-appearing skin surface.

4. It can improve skin elasticity.

Step 3: Removal of abnormal pigment and blood vessels

The accumulation of pigment (brown spots) and the proliferation of visible superficial blood vessels (red spots) on the surface of the skin are the skin's inflammatory response to years of damaging UV sunlight injury and other toxic injuries, both from the environment and from within our own bodies. These changes are classic signs of facial skin ageing. Removal of these blemishes imparts the following rejuvenation effects.

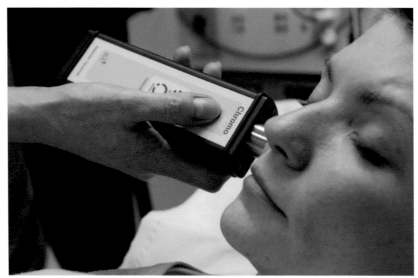

Improvements can be made by removing uneven pigment from the skin.

1. A homogeneous, even, unblemished, youthful skin appearance and colour.

2. Removal of atypical damaged inflammatory lesions that may in the future evolve into more serious and extensive abnormal facial lesions such as actinic keratoses, possible precursors to skin cancer.

Step 4: Relaxation of the muscles of facial expression

As discussed earlier, continued contraction of the muscles of facial expression throughout life results in the development of the lines of facial expression. These lines, known commonly as crow's feet, frown lines, worry lines and bunny lines, are noticeable facial wrinkles that impart a characteristic aged appearance to the face. Any effective facial rejuvenation programme must address these significant Type II facial ageing changes. Relaxation of the muscles of facial expression will have the following effects.

1. Remove or soften the crow's feet, frown lines, worry lines and bunny lines.

2. Prevent the recurrence of these lines once facial rejuvenation has been achieved and avoid renewed Type II facial ageing changes caused by these muscles.

Step 5: Filling of deep facial lines and contour deformities

The combination of dermal atrophy, subcutaneous fat loss, loss of elasticity and sagging facial soft-tissue structures creates several different facial deformities that are classically associated with facial

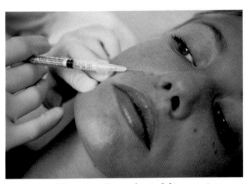

ageing. Inferior migration, thinning and lengthening of the upper lip, the appearance of deep lines or depressions in the facial skin (the nasal–labial fold and marionette lines), the tear trough deformity and the 'dark circle' beneath the lower eyelid are examples that impart a very aged appearance to the facial skin. Improvement in the appearance of these deformities requires volume

Filling in deep facial lines gives a smoother appearance.

replacement that will result in the following.

1. Softening of the appearance of these defects by plumping the depressions and lessening the shadow created by them.

2. Filling or plumping the lip to a fuller, more youthful appearance.

3. Filling depressions caused by dermal and subcutaneous fat atrophy or the descent of soft tissues to an inferior location.

Step 6: Tightening of the facial skin

The loss of skin elasticity secondary to damage to dermal collagen and elastin, and atrophy of the subcutaneous fat and, to a lesser extent, bony atrophy (at advanced ages) result in a downward migration or sagging of the facial skin. Clinically, this results in several anatomical facial changes associated with an aged facial appearance, commonly called jowls (loose skin folds along the jaw), turkey neck or turkey wattle (loose skin folds on the neck and beneath the chin), sagging cheek and sagging eyebrow, which can obscure the vision if it overhangs the eye significantly. While steps 1–5 address almost all of the Type I superficial skin ageing changes, the dynamic Type II facial-expression-induced changes, and many of the Type II volumetric facial ageing changes, the descent of the facial skin envelope resulting from the loss of elasticity and major volumetric loss are not yet fully addressed. Tightening of the facial skin envelope is required for effective facial rejuvenation in patients who have facial skin sufficiently aged in appearance to demonstrate the anatomical changes described above in this paragraph. For these individuals, tightening of the facial skin will provide the following.

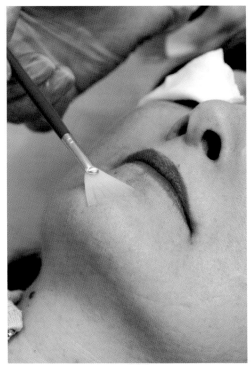

Tightening the facial skin can counteract loss of elasticity.

❧ Restoration of the cheek skin to a higher, more youthful position over the cheekbone or zygomatic arch.

❧ Restoration of the high point of the eyebrow to a position at least 1 centimetre above the supraorbital rim (the upper brow bone).

❧ Restoration of a smooth jaw line extending from the chin to the angle of the jawbone, which lies below the ear.

❧ Restoration of a clean neckline approximating a right-angle at the intersection of a line extending from below the chin to the thyroid cartilage (Adam's apple) and from the thyroid cartilage down to the suprasternal notch (the top of the breastbone).

The six-step programme in action — how it's done

Effective facial rejuvenation requires the help of an *experienced* **accredited physician** who has the ability to provide you with all components of the six-step programme. More importantly, the physician must understand how to apply the various therapies to your unique face and in the proper sequence. Because this programme is new and not widely understood by doctors, I am providing you with the specifics of how it works. In this way, you will have the knowledge required to make certain you are receiving proper treatment. You will be an educated consumer, and making you an educated consumer is what this book is about.

Programme preparation — preliminary steps

Before we begin our therapeutic action plan for rejuvenating your face, it is essential that your nutritional and lifestyle choices and your daily skin-care routine be optimised for the facial rejuvenation process. In Chapter 4 we discussed the importance of diet, exercise, stress management and the avoidance of sun and other harmful environmental factors in preventing facial ageing. It just does not make sense to embark on a rigorous programme to reverse facial ageing changes if you do not have the preventative and basic corrective practices as part of your daily routine. Furthermore, for those of you who have very early minimal ageing changes, instituting these preliminary steps is the best way to avoid the expense and effort required for the full

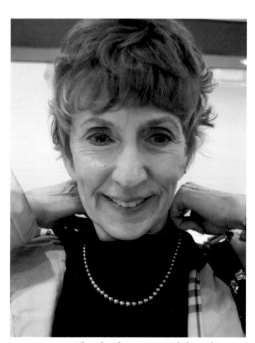

Think about your lifestyle choices before embarking on therapeutic action.

six-step programme. Programme preparation focuses on three important areas of your health:

1. lifestyle and fitness

2. diet

3. your customised daily skin-care programme.

Lifestyle and fitness

In Chapter 4 I stressed the importance of avoiding free-radical-producing agents that damage collagen and age your skin. Let's review the obvious ones again.

To promote healthy skin and avoid ageing changes the following guidelines are important.

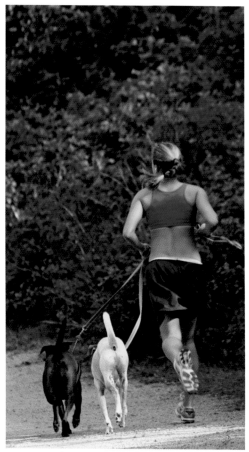

Regular exercise should be something you enjoy.

❦ Avoid excessive sun exposure – always wear sun block, sunglasses and sun-protective gear such as a visor or hat when you are exposed to the sun.

❦ Do not smoke cigarettes.

❦ Avoid excessive alcohol consumption.

❦ Start an exercise programme that includes resistance and aerobic training.

❦ Begin seriously working on stress management techniques – remember, cortisol released when you are stressed destroys the collagen in your skin.

❦ Work on your spiritual self.

Diet

A healthy diet rich in anti-inflammatory foods and antioxidants is important for skin health and is essential for the success of your facial rejuvenation programme.

Avoid:

* refined starches,

* sugars,

* saturated fats,

* animal fats.

Consume:

* anti-inflammatory foods such as omega-3 oils, salmon, sardines and other cold-water fish,

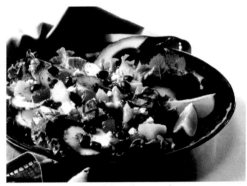

Choose a healthy diet rich on antioxidants.

* soy instead of dairy,

* foods high in fibre,

* whole grains,

* fruits,

* vegetables, especially bright-coloured ones.

Important supplements

* Flaxseed powder (2 tbsp/day).

* Antioxidant vitamins (see Chapter 4).

Your customised daily skin-care routine

I try to make certain that all my patients are on an optimal preventative and/or corrective skin-care programme before starting any advanced facial rejuvenation therapy. Following my initial evaluation, my **aesthetician** and I decide which programme is most appropriate for the patient's unique face and skin type.

It is helpful to classify your skin into one of four common categories. Everyone's facial skin is different and one person's facial skin may fit into more than one category, but try to decide which category most closely resembles the changes you see in your facial skin. The four categories are as follows.

1. *Hyperpigmented skin.* Hyperpigmented skin is characterised by the presence of brown spots or patchy brown or reddish brown areas on the face, most typically in the areas that receive the most sun exposure.

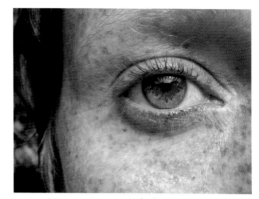

Hyperpigmented skin is characterised by brown spots.

2. *Dry skin with wrinkles.* Dry skin is typically thin and fair and often has fine lines and wrinkles at an earlier age than people with darker, more oily facial skin.

3. *Oily skin with enlarged pores.* People with oily skin often have enlarged pores and are prone to acne outbreaks, especially during periods of hormonal fluctuations.

4. *Sensitive skin or rosacea.* People with sensitive skin and those with rosacea have skin that is easily irritated and often have patchy redness and small blood vessels on the skin surface.

Those of you who have a combination of the characteristics described above should focus your skin care first on the predominant characteristic. After you see improvement in the predominant characteristic, switch to or add the regimen directed towards the remaining problem area.

Start slowly. More is not better, and skin care that is too aggressive will cause irritation and negative results. As you progress, with the advice of your doctor and aesthetician, you may be more aggressive.

The products listed in Table 5.1 are the ones I use in my practice. They are sold only in doctors' offices because they contain a higher percentage of active ingredients than those sold over the counter in department stores or chemists. I use products made by La Roche-Posay, Innovative Skincare™ and Obagi® because I have found them to be very effective and well liked by my patients. I have no commercial interest in these products. There are many other fine products available, and I suggest that you rely on the advice of your own physician. Alternatively, if you have products you are happy

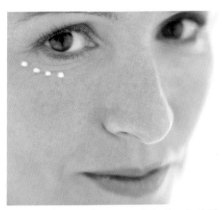

Caring for your skin is vital if you want to maintain youthful good looks.

with, substitute them for those in the chart below. The important point is to follow a daily morning and evening cycle of:

❧ cleanse,

❧ tone,

❧ eye cream,

❧ correct,

❧ moisturise (a.m.)/ exfoliate (p.m.),

❧ protect.

Table 5.1 Daily skin-care routine. Identify your skin type and follow morning and night routines

a.m.	Cleanse	Tone	Eye cream	Correct	Moisturise	Protect
Hyperpigmentation	Purifying cleanser	Conditioning Solution[1]	Eye Complex[2]	EpiQuin˜ or Glyquin˜	Hydraphase[1] (if needed)	SPF30 with moisturiser
Dry skin and wrinkles	Micro-exfoliating scrub[1]	Conditioning Solution[1] (if tolerated)	Eye Complex[2]	Super Serum[2]	Moisturising Complex[2]	SPF30 with moisturiser
Oily skin and enlarged pores	Effaclar gel solution[1]	Conditioning Solution[1]	Eye Complex[2]	Effaclar K1	No	SPF30 with moisturiser
Sensitive skin and rosacea	Toleriane Dermo-cleanser[1] or Toleriane Foaming Cleanser[1]	Gentle Soothing Toner[1]	Eye Complex[2]	ProHeal Serum[2]	Moisturising Complex[2]	SPF30 with moisturiser

p.m.	Cleanse	Tone	Eye cream	Correct	Exfoliant	Protect
Hyperpigmentation	Purifying Cleanser[1]	Conditioning Solution[1]	Eye Complex[2]	EpiQuin˜ or Glyquin˜	Active Serum[2]	Moisturising Complex[2]
Dry skin and wrinkles	Micro-exfoliating Scrub[1]	Conditioning Solution[1] (if tolerated)	Eye Complex[2]	Retin-A˜, Tazorac˜ or Avage˜	Firming Complex[2]	Moisturising Complex[2]
Oily skin and enlarged pores	Effaclar Gel[1]	Conditioning Solution[1]	Eye Complex[2]	Retin-A˜, Tazorac˜ or Avage˜	Effaclar K[1]	Toleriane Facial Fluid[1]
Sensitive skin and rosacea	Toleriane Dermo-cleanser[1] or Toleriane Foaming Cleanser[1]	Gentle Soothing Toner[1]	Eye Complex[2]	Renova˜ or OTC Retinol	No	Toleriane Facial Cream[2]

1. La Roche-Posay/BioMedic˜ 2. Innovative Skincare˜

Step 1: Exfoliation

I start all of my patients on an exfoliation routine consisting of topical exfoliating creams and microdermabrasion or superficial **chemical peels** with glycolic or salicylic acid. The chemical peels are **'no down time' procedures**: you leave the office a little pink, but with a refreshed glow. The exfoliating creams I use are Retin-A" and Tazarotine", although for patients with sensitive skin I use vitamin C topically.

For patients with more severe ageing changes, I use a deeper form of exfoliation called **MicroLaserPeel**" (see photographs below). This goes deeper than a microdermabrasion and is more effective, but you leave the office quite red and it takes 4–6 days for your skin to look normal. This is a great improvement over **laser resurfacing**, which goes much deeper and requires many weeks of recovery. CO_2 Lite", a new feature on the UltraPulse Encore" CO_2 laser resurfacing machine, is another exciting new exfoliation technique. Many physicians use deeper chemical peels with trichloroacetic acid (TCA), but I prefer the MicroLaserPeel" because of its accuracy and reliability. The Obagi Blue Peel" is another good alternative.

Exfoliation not only removes dead skin, but also lightens pigment and stimulates the production of new collagen growth in the deeper layers of the skin. I start with exfoliation because several of the

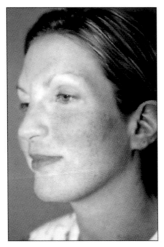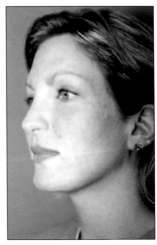

Before (left) and after (right) a 40-micron MicroLaserPeel".

subsequent steps work better after it. More importantly, the abnormal blood vessels may be more apparent after exfoliation and it would therefore be an error to treat the blood vessels first.

Step 2: Stimulate new collagen formation

After deep exfoliation, this is the most important step for the removal of static facial wrinkles and fine lines. This step is also the most time consuming and tedious and requires patience on your part. There is no quick, non-surgical way to remove visible facial wrinkles. Although laser resurfacing can quickly and effectively remove facial wrinkles, I consider it to be a surgical procedure, and the prolonged recovery and **down time** make it unacceptable for most people.

Although the deep exfoliation and topical creams mentioned above stimulate new collagen production, additional stimulation is required. Several new laser techniques, intense pulsed light (IPL) and **radiofrequency** machines can stimulate the skin to form new collagen in the deeper layers without damaging the skin surface. These techniques are called **non-ablative**, meaning that they do not remove the surface skin cells, as is done in laser resurfacing, which is an **ablative** technique. Consequently, these non-ablative techniques are 'no down time' procedures, which means that after a treatment your skin is pink but recovers quickly, within hours.

The non-ablative laser, IPL and radiofrequency techniques work by a sophisticated heating of the deep layers of the skin causing it to respond by forming new collagen. The exact mechanism is explained in Chapter 8, 'High-tech facial rejuvenation'.

There are many different brands of machines that can perform non-ablative stimulation of collagen formation, often called **photo** (or foto) **rejuvenation**. I prefer one called Laser Genesis™ because it involves no contact with the skin and therefore there is minimal discomfort for the patient as well as minimal down time and skin injury. IPL is also effective in patients who have a lot of pigment and abnormal blood vessels, but it delivers more heat in direct contact with the skin and thus slightly more discomfort and redness for the patient, and therefore must be used with caution and only by someone who is trained and experienced in its use.

Collagen stimulation is a lengthy process. An effective result that you can see in the mirror, i.e. fewer wrinkles, requires at least 5–7 treatments, and 5–7 months for the benefit to be visible. However, it took 30–40 years for the wrinkles to form, so removal in 7 months without surgery and down time is pretty good (see photgraphs below).

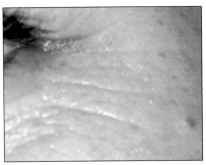 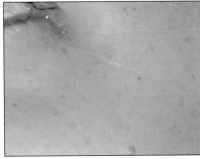

Before (left) and after (right) Laser Genesis™ treatments to stimulate new collagen formation in the crow's feet area.

Step 3: Removal of abnormal pigment and blood vessels

Although creams and exfoliation can remove many light brown spots, and the lasers and IPL used in Step 2 remove small vessels, more aggressive therapy is needed for the removal of darker pigment and brown spots and larger vessels. There are many non-ablative lasers available for this purpose. Although these lasers are non-ablative, they do leave a reddish mark that is visible for a day or two but easily covered with make-up. I have used a laser called the VersaPulse™ for many years, which works very well (see photographs below), but new VersaPulse™ lasers are so expensive that they are rarely manufactured today.

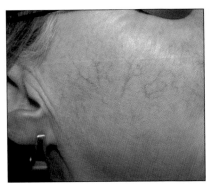 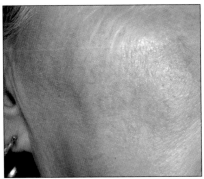

Before (left) and after (right) laser removal of superficial blood vessels.

A newer laser called the CoolGlide™ is very effective for larger blood vessels. The IPL is currently the best option for combined pigment and smaller blood vessels that appear as a flush similar to rosacea (see photographs below).

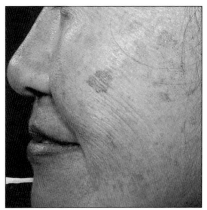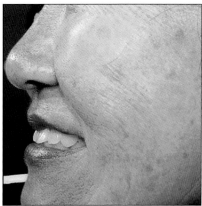

Before (left) and after (right) pigment removal with intense pulsed light (IPL).

The above therapies are effective and results are visible in about 6 weeks. Two or three treatments are usually needed.

Step 4: Relaxation of muscles of facial expression

Botox™ is a revolutionary new drug that effectively removes dynamic lines and wrinkles caused by the muscles of facial expression. The frown lines, worry lines, crow's feet and bunny lines may all be lessened or removed by the injection of Botox™. It may also lessen lipstick lines (fine wrinkles around the lips), but only small amounts can be used, otherwise the lips will be weakened.

There are several new 'peptides', for example acetyl hexapeptide-3, which, when applied topically as a cream, are reported to have a Botox™-like effect in reducing fine lines. Eventually these agents will be perfected and be more effective and will possibly make Botox™ injections unnecessary; however, convincing studies of their effectiveness are not yet available. For now, I use Botox™.

You can read more about how these muscle-relaxing, wrinkle-removing agents work in Chapter 7, '"No down time" facial anti-ageing procedures'.

Step 5: Fill deep facial lines and contour deformities

Soft-tissue fillers such as Radiesse™, Restylane™, your own fat and other fillers can be injected into the skin beneath a deep facial line to plump and camouflage it. Restylane™ may also be used to plump the ageing lip and to fill contour deformities caused by facial ageing.

These fillers are temporary and the process must be repeated every 6 months to a year. Fat injections can last longer and, if done properly, may not need to be repeated. Remember, however, that the filler techniques are a camouflage, not a correction.

Step 6: Skin tightening

Skin tightening is a very important component of any facial rejuvenation process. Prior to the past year or two, a face-lift was the only option for tightening facial skin. However, new technologies using **infrared** and radiofrequency energy are showing promising results as non-surgical skin-tightening methods.

Two of these methods, Thermage™, which uses radiofrequency energy, and Titan™, an infrared device, have been used for 3 years and results are improving. These methods are not non-surgical face-lifts, as so often advertised, so do not be misled. They can, however, tighten skin by as much as 30 per cent in properly selected patients. There have been complications with Thermage™, consisting of

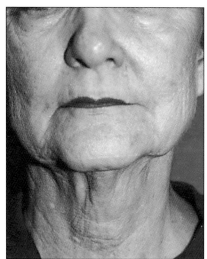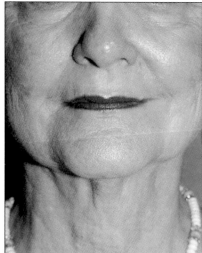

*Before (left) and after (right) treatment of neck and jaw
skin laxity with Titan™.*

97

depressions in certain areas of the facial skin, so your doctor's expertise and experience in the use of these machines are very important.

As with other non-surgical facial rejuvenation techniques, skin tightening requires multiple treatments and it takes time to see the final result, often 5–6 months. As with the other laser and photo techniques mentioned above, skin tightening is achieved by stimulating the deeper layers of the skin to remodel and form new collagen.

Non-surgical skin tightening is most useful for younger patients who are beginning to develop loose skin in the neck and cheek and along the jaw-line. Severe facial sagging in older patients can be improved, but the results will be less impressive.

The treatments take time – although a new device called FACES™ (functional aspiration controlled electrothermal stimulation) by Lumenis™ is reported to take less time – and technique is very important. For an in-depth discussion of how skin tightening works, see Chapter 8, 'High-tech facial rejuvenation'.

Finally, don't be misled by advertisements for non-surgical face-lifts called the Feather Lift™, Thread Lift™, Contour Lift™ etc. These are all *surgical* procedures that carry all the inherent risks of a surgical procedure, and results for many of them have been disappointing. You can read more about these procedures in Chapter 7, '"No down time" facial anti-ageing procedures'.

The 6-Step Non-surgical Facial Rejuvenation Program® is a carefully structured method for the application of revolutionary new techniques to obtain effective non-surgical rejuvenation. This programme takes time, but the results are visible and real after about 7 months – people using creams and diets during the same time period end up with no visible difference. Remember, it took a lifetime for your face to age. Does it make sense that this damage can be reversed overnight? Of course not.

The non-surgical facial rejuvenation programme is expensive. These new technologies are costly, and of course you need to be treated by a qualified physician. However, with my six-step programme you get what you pay for: facial rejuvenation without the risk, discomfort and expense of surgery. If you add up the cost of your skin creams, facials, fad diets and spa visits, and save this money for the six-step programme, many of you will be very close to covering the cost. For those of you who are already having facial rejuvenation treatments in a doctor's office, the six-step programme will produce better, more effective results and save you money.

Table 5.2 summarises my 6-Step Non-surgical Facial Rejuvenation Program®. The individual methods are discussed in detail in the following chapters.

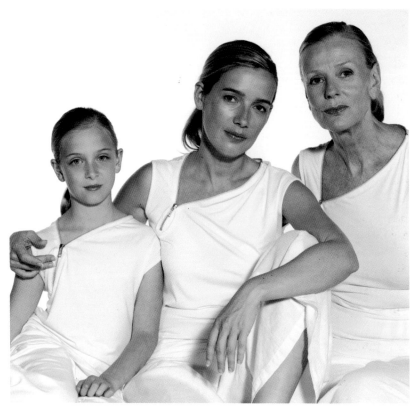

You can make informed choices about how to defy the generation gap!

Table 5.2 Dr Seckel's six-step programme

Anti-ageing	Ageing change treated	Treatments available
Step 1: Exfoliation	Revitalise aged dry skin	Microdermabrasion; topical creams; MicroPeel™; MicroLaserPeel™; CO_2 Lite™
Step 2: Regenerate dermal collagen and elastin	Plump and firm skin	Lasers; IPL; topical creams; exfoliation
Step 3: Remove brown spots and telangiectasias	Remove blemishes	Lasers; IPL; topical creams; exfoliation
Step 4: Relax muscles of facial expression	Correct worry lines, frown lines, crow's feet, bunny lines	Botox™; topical creams
Step 5: Camouflage deep facial lines	Camouflage nasal–labial fold lines and marionette lines	Fillers
Step 6: Tighten facial skin	Correct loose skin and wrinkles	Laser resurfacing; collagen remodelling; non-surgical tightening (Titan™, Thermage™, FACES™)

6 Magical potions – the fountain of youth

Topical skin creams

Millions of pounds (more than $20 billion a year in the USA), are spent on skin creams to prevent or reverse facial ageing. Most of that money is wasted. The majority of the non-prescription anti-ageing creams do not work.

The most important thing I want you to remember as you read this chapter is that *the only two treatments that have been approved by the US Food and Drug Administration (FDA) as effective for reversing facial ageing changes are Retin-A™ and Tazarotine™, two prescription creams, and laser resurfacing.* Laser resurfacing is, of course, a surgical procedure.

The competitive marketing of anti-ageing skin creams has created a confounding array of products. As Dr Klingman (the pioneer who developed Retin-A™) put it, 'We have a marketplace that is absolutely crazy and the consumer is left to do her own personal clinical trial to see what works.'[1] The US FDA requires labelling on prescription creams other than Retin-A™ to state in bold print: 'These products do not remove or prevent wrinkles, repair **sun-damaged skin**, reverse ageing due to sun or restore your more youthful skin'. Certainly, FDA approval often lags behind the development of promising new therapies, but the FDA waits for scientifically valid clinical studies before it grants approval.

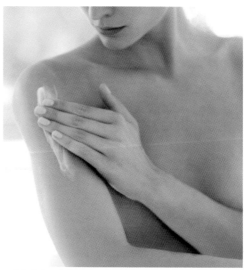

Moisturising your skin regularly will help to keep it supple.

So what can you do? Consult a reputable doctor who specialises in facial ageing, a **dermatologist** or a plastic surgeon who is informed and up to date on this subject. Don't rely on what you read in beauty magazines, what you hear on talk shows or from the charming salesperson at the cosmetic counter. Set the pop-up ad. controls on your computer so you won't be bombarded with that annoying array of false promises that are designed to pull you in and take your money!

The worst offenders are the **infomercials**. Think about that word 'infomercial'. It is used to sucker you in. These are commercials designed to sell you a product. They add the prefix 'info' instead of 'com' to make you think they are providing you with valid information. Listen to what they're saying. Do they provide you with a reference reporting a clinical trial published in a medical journal? Of course not, because there is none!

I saw an infomercial on TV in which a beautiful movie star was touting the advantages of a miracle cream that was purported to be 'better than Botox™'. Do you realise that such spokespersons are paid for their statements and often have never used the product? In my opinion, nowhere is this misleading type of advertising more pervasive than in the field of anti-ageing creams and solutions. Why? Because this field is so 'hot'. These entrepreneurs have read the data on the huge population of ageing baby boomers who do not want to grow old, and we are ripe for the picking.

Please read this chapter carefully, and only use products for which there are some scientifically proven data to support their use. In the discussion below, I differentiate between claims made for agents for which there are clinical studies to back them up and those that may make intuitive sense but do not yet have the science to justify them. The most effective, proven skin creams and solutions require a doctor's prescription. Does this surprise you? I doubt it.

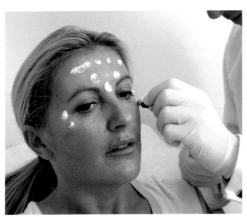

The appropriate topical creams can have a beneficial effect.

How do topical creams, gels, ointments and solutions correct ageing changes?

Topical agents can reverse facial ageing changes in the following ways.

❧ Exfoliating or removing dead epithelial cells from the skin surface.

❧ Promoting the growth of new epithelial cells.

❧ Halting the production of pigment, which causes brown spots.

❧ Stimulating the production of new collagen in the dermis.

❧ Blocking the production of enzymes that break down or destroy collagen.

❧ Delivering antioxidants or free-radical scavengers to the skin.

Remember, these effects occur at a sub-microscopic cellular level. Don't expect visible, drastic or immediate results. The changes produced by skin creams are subtle and are noticed only after 6 months or a year of continued daily use. Claims of a 'face-lift in a jar' or a cream that causes 'immediate plumping of the skin or lips' are nonsense, unless, of course, you have an **allergic reaction** to the cream or it is an irritant!

Retin-A™

This chemical, also known as tretinoin, is a by-product of vitamin A synthesis and a member of a key family of skin-care medications called the retinoids. Retinoids regulate the growth of the epidermis, inhibit the formation of cancer, decrease inflammation and improve immune function. Retin-A™ is a prescription drug; you cannot buy it at the beauty counter. In cream form, it has been clinically proven to improve the epithelium by stimulating the development and growth of new epithelial

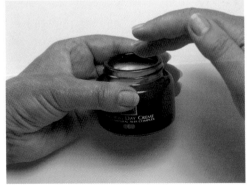

Retin-A™ *is a by-product of vitamin A.*

103

cells to replace the old and damaged ones. It also stimulates new collagen production, prevents collagen breakdown and lessens pigmentation.[2] Why would you want to use anything else?

To improve its anti-ageing effectiveness, Retin-A™ can be mixed with hydroquinone 4 per cent, a bleaching cream, to enhance the removal of pigment or brown spots. In addition, when used in conjunction with microdermabrasion (which is discussed in more detail in the next chapter), Retin-A™'s penetration and effectiveness are enhanced.

Retin-A™ is too irritating to the skin for many people, however. Also, it can sensitise your skin to the sun, so it is essential to wear sun block and skin protection (such as a hat and large sunglasses) while using it. Newer, less-irritating compounds are Renova™ and Retin-A Micro™. Retin-A™ comes in different strengths: 0.01 per cent, 0.025 per cent, 0.05 per cent, and 0.1 per cent. I typically start patients on 0.025 per cent to see if they can tolerate the product well, and if they can, I gradually increase the strength. Tazorac™

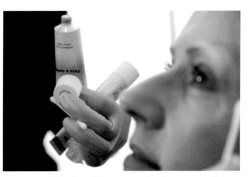

Trained cosmetologists use the most effective topical products.

and Avage™ (available in the UK on prescription as Zorac™), two other products containing Tazarotine™ (a retinoid that has been very effective for treating psoriasis and acne), are now approved for their anti-ageing effects.

Retinols

Retinols are available as over-the-counter products, no prescription necessary. Although their effectiveness is a matter of controversy among dermatologists, these compounds, once applied, are converted in your skin to retinoesters and small quantities of tretinoin. Combining retinol 0.3 per cent with hydroquinone 4 per cent (EpiQuin™) is effective in resolving fine lines and pigment and improving skin texture.[3] Retinols are not as strong as Retin-A™ and therefore can be used by many people who cannot tolerate the stronger product.

Alpha-hydroxy acids

The alpha-hydroxy acids (AHAs) – glycolic acid and lactic acid – are derived from fruit and milk sugars. The AHA most commonly used is glycolic acid, which is widely added to over-the-counter skin creams and used by aestheticians and doctors to perform skin peels to reverse skin-ageing damage and pigmentation.

The AHAs produce exfoliation and stimulate the production of new collagen in the dermis, so they are a valuable component of most anti-ageing skin-care regimens. A recent study also showed that glycolic acid treatment of the skin increased the hyaluronic acid (HA) content of both the epidermis and dermis, a very exciting finding since, as we know, loss of HA is an important cause of dryness in aged skin.[4]

Don't let their benign origins fool you though! The AHAs can be very irritating. There are estimated to be thousands of adverse reactions to AHA-containing products each year, reactions that can include redness, swelling of the eyes, rash, itching and skin discoloration.[5] Stronger solutions of the AHAs are used by doctors to produce a chemical peel, which blisters or removes the epithelium and irritates the dermis in order to encourage more new collagen production.

Skin-care products containing glycolic or lactic acid that are sold over the counter contain, at most, only 10 per cent of the AHA. Trained **cosmetologists** may use products that contain 20–30 per cent AHA, and doctors may use products with as much as 50–70 per cent, but at these concentrations a deep chemical peel is produced.

I frequently use AHAs, in both prescription and non-prescription forms, for patients who cannot tolerate Retin-A˜. The Cosmetic Ingredient Review Panel[5] concludes that the AHAs glycolic and lactic acid are safe for the consumer when:

❀ the AHA concentration is 10 per cent or less,

❀ the **pH** is 3.5 or higher,

❀ the product contains sunscreen or the label clearly recommends the use of sunscreen.

Vitamin C – L-ascorbic acid

Vitamin C is an important antioxidant, which, in the form of L-ascorbic acid (also known as vitamin C ester) can be applied topically to the skin. When vitamin C ester is put in a lipophilic (fat-loving) solution, it may be possible to deliver it directly to the skin.[6] As you will remember, the walls of skin cells contain fat, and the vitamin C ester must be in a solution that can penetrate this fatty barrier to get into the skin to have an effect.

Vitamin C ester has multiple anti-ageing effects: it's a free-radical scavenger, it promotes new collagen formation and it actively protects skin from the ageing effects of ultraviolet (UV) radiation in sunlight, above and beyond the benefit provided by sun block. Its effect is enhanced by the addition of vitamin E7. I frequently use vitamin C preparations for patients who cannot tolerate Retin-A™, and for patients with rosacea or other inflammatory skin conditions for whom Retin-A™ is too irritating.

Vitamin E (tocopherols and tocotrienols)

You will recall from Chapters 3 and 4 that vitamin E is one of the most powerful antioxidants and has been shown to be beneficial in combating both heart disease and cancer. Vitamin E also plays a role in protecting the skin from ageing damage caused by the sun[7, 8] when used in combination with vitamin C in sun block. Traditionally, vitamin E has been taken orally along with other antioxidants, but topical solutions containing vitamin E have recently become available. Many new prescription anti-ageing creams have vitamin E and other antioxidant vitamins in their formulas.

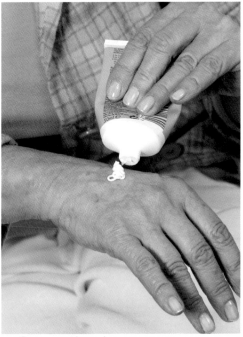

Some anti-ageing creams are effective moisturisers.

Alpha-lipoic acid

Recently, there has been much interest in the antioxidant alpha-lipoic acid (ALA) as a useful supplement for preventing facial ageing.[9] Most of the oft-quoted studies have in fact been done on rats, so definitive evidence of the usefulness of ALA in humans awaits further research. One clinical study in humans has been published, which suggests that topical application of ALA can reverse textural changes in the facial skin associated with ageing.[10] Whether these changes are the result of epithelial cell regeneration and new collagen formation or of some other direct effect on the skin (such as improving moisture content or swelling) needs to be determined by microscopic studies of skin biopsies.

Coenzyme Q10 (ubiquinone, idebenone)

As discussed in Chapter 4, coenzyme Q10 is important in cellular metabolism and acts as an antioxidant to protect cell membranes from damage by free radicals. As we've learned, the results of clinical studies into the effectiveness of coenzyme Q10 in humans are equivocal. Although coenzyme Q10 is being sold as a component of some topical solutions, I can find no scientifically controlled clinical studies in which it has been shown to be useful as a topical agent.

Recently, there has been a great deal of publicity about a synthetic analogue of coenzyme Q10 called idebenone. In laboratory experiments, idebenone has proven to be a more powerful antioxidant than coenzyme Q10. One early, but unpublished, clinical trial involving 28 patients and provided by the company that makes Prevage™ (a cream containing idebenone) reports encouraging results.

Polyenylphosphatidyl choline

Polyenylphosphatidyl choline (PPC), a phospholipid (fat) with antioxidant properties, has been touted as an effective emollient and anti-ageing cream.[9] To my knowledge, the main therapeutic use of this agent documented in the scientific literature is in alcoholic liver disease in rats.[11] Therefore, if you are a non-rat, I would wait for controlled clinical studies in humans before pinning anti-ageing hopes on this topical preparation! PPC may well be a good moisturiser, but there are many others available, some of which are more appealing to me on a scientific basis (see 'Hyaluronic acid' below).

Dimethylaminoethanol – 'face-lift in a jar'?

Remember what I wrote about things that are too good to be true? Dimethylaminoethanol (DMAE) has been recommended as a treatment for Alzheimer's disease, tardive dyskinesia (a movement disorder related to Parkinson's disease) and attention deficit disorder. However, controlled clinical studies have failed to show a demonstrable benefit of this agent in any of these conditions. Why would you expect it to give you a face-lift?

DMEA is a precursor of choline, which is a component of acetylcholine, the chemical released from nerves to make the facial muscles contract (tighten). The theory is that if you apply DMAE, choline synthesis will be increased, leading to increased production of acetylcholine, which will result in contraction (or tightening) of your facial muscles and tightening of your skin.

One recent report[12] of a split-face study in which one side of the face was treated with DMAE and the other side was not treated suggested that topical DMEA did in fact tighten one side of the face.

The proposed mechanism of this tightening is contraction of the facial muscles. Do you remember from Chapter 2 what causes frown lines, worry lines and crow's feet? The answer is, of course, muscle contraction! We block the action of acetylcholine with Botox™ to *weaken* muscle contraction and get rid of facial lines. Furthermore, what causes the skin to sag is loss of elasticity, not loss of muscle contraction. It seems to me that the 'face-lift in a jar' and Botox™ work against each other. Perhaps you can use them both together.

When taken orally, DMAE can have serious side effects, including worsening of depression and schizophrenia.[13] Personally, I think I would go for the face-lift!

Perhaps this compound will be used in the future to firm the skin by some not yet clearly understood mechanism, but at present I am sceptical. I can assure you that DMAE is not a face-lift in a jar, which is a preposterous claim.

Acetyl hexapeptide-3 – 'better than Botox™'?

The shameless hyperbole of the vendors of anti-ageing creams casts a sorrowful shadow on what might be a promising new drug.

According to the companies that sell products containing acetyl hexapeptide-3, it is a highly sophisticated, genetically engineered protein designed to block the release of acetylcholine from nerve endings. This is a mechanism for muscle relaxation similar to that of Botox", but it occurs at a much smaller site, on the cell membrane of the nerve terminal.

Manufacturers of products containing acetyl hexapeptide-3 claim that this chemical can be delivered through the skin in the form of a topical cream, and slowly and minimally relax the facial muscles and reduce wrinkles. Some claim that this chemical prolongs the effects of Botox".

Unfortunately, the only article offering a clinical study showing significant results was on a website that offered to sell you their product, but failed to reference a publication for their study (www.cremedevie.com). Several creams, among them Avotox", StriVectin-SD", Serum XL" and Creme de Vie", are claimed to contain acetyl hexapeptide-3 and to remove wrinkles by the above mechanism.

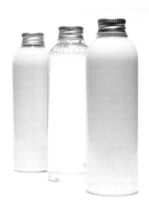

Again, an extensive search of the credible scientific literature failed to substantiate these claims. Perhaps this newly manufactured protein is so new that studies have not been published, but if that is

After the age of 50, it becomes more important than ever to moisturise your skin.

the case, I question whether or not they should be selling it to you, the consumer. Perhaps controlled clinical trials will be done to prove or disprove the effectiveness of these new creams.

However, the concept is very exciting, and if the claims are substantiated by controlled clinical studies, this truly will be a revolutionary new product.

Palmitoyl pentapeptide

Palmitoyl pentapeptide (also known as palmitoyl oligopeptide) is a new skin rejuvenation compound. Proponents claim that it is at least as effective against wrinkles as retinol but does not cause skin irritation, a common side effect of retinoids.

Chemically speaking, palmitoyl pentapeptide is a relatively small molecule (five amino acids linked together and attached to a fatty acid) that is structurally related to the precursor of collagen type I (procollagen type I). Researchers found that when added to a culture of fibroblasts (the key collagen-producing skin cells), palmitoyl pentapeptide stimulated the synthesis of the key constituents of the skin matrix: collagen, elastin and glucosaminoglycans.

So far, the clinical data are encouraging. One study demonstrated that palmitoyl pentapeptide was as effective as retinol in repairing sun-damaged skin, but without the side effects. So, palmitoyl pentapeptide, with its good safety profile, may be worth a try. It may also be considered as a non-irritating fallback option for people who develop skin irritation in response to retinoids or alpha-hydroxy acids.

Hyaluronic acid

As mentioned in Chapter 2, HA is a crucial moisturising and nutrition-providing substance found throughout the skin. By the age of 50, we have lost much of this valuable skin component. HA has recently been in the news as a filler to inject into the skin to correct wrinkles (see the next chapter). What I am discussing here is the use of HA in skin creams. Widely used as a humectant (or moisturiser) in skin creams, HA is excellent in this role.

Whether or not topically applied HA is actually taken up by the dermis and contributes to the total skin content of HA is unknown. In my opinion it is unlikely, in view of the fact that the very pure forms of HA that we inject into the skin as fillers are biodegraded in a matter of 6–9 months and injections have to be repeated to maintain the correction of wrinkles and deep facial lines. If we could restore the HA content of our skin, improvement in moisture content, firmness and suppleness would result.

I think it is unlikely that any cream, gel or other topical agent can restore the HA lost by ageing. Oestrogen has been reported to increase HA synthesis in the skin, but the dangers of oestrogen replacement outweigh this potential benefit. Creams containing HA are wonderful moisturisers, but I would not recommend you pay a premium expecting the cream to reverse ageing by regenerating the HA content of your skin.

Bleaching agents

Hydroquinone 4 per cent and kojic acid are two very useful skin **bleaching agents**. Superficial pigmentation, a Type I ageing skin change, can be lightened by using these bleaching creams, especially when they are used in combination with a retinoid such as Retin-A™ or retinol. Pigment removal is also enhanced when these agents are used in conjunction with exfoliation such as microdermabrasion (see Chapter 7).

Hydroquinone should be stopped after 6 months of use, as there is risk of **hypopigmentation** with prolonged use. It may be used again after a rest period of 3–6 months. Three months on and 3 months off is another acceptable way to use hydroquinone.

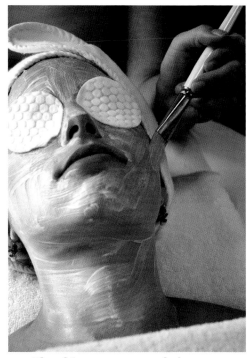

Bleaching creams can help improve superficial skin pigmentation.

Summary

In summary, I urge you to go back and read the first few paragraphs of this chapter. The cosmetic and pharmaceutical industries have become incredibly sophisticated in their marketing approaches. They know our generation is informed and well educated and demands to understand the science behind the claims they make about their products.

Seriously reviewing this topic was an incredible eye-opener for me. When you carefully review the claims made for many of the anti-ageing products, it becomes apparent that there are very few hard data and few scientifically controlled clinical studies to support the incredible claims that are made about most, if not all, of these new 'miracle' products.

What's happening is this: an exciting new theory or very early discovery is produced, packaged and marketed to you as if the anti-ageing benefits are proven facts. They are not. You need to be an informed consumer and, more than ever, you need the advice of a knowledgeable doctor to help you sort through the confusing array of claims and counter-claims. I have tried to give you a good review of this topic as I understand it, and my findings are summarised in Table 6.1.

Table 6.1 Anti-ageing products

Product	Action	Effect	Proven to work	Brand names	Dr Seckel recommends
Tretinoin	Promotes growth of new epithelium; promotes new collagen	Helps remove fine lines and pigment; improves the look of the skin	Yes	Retin-A"	Yes
Tazarotine	Promotes growth of new epithelium; promotes new collagen	Helps remove fine lines and pigment; improves the look of the skin	Yes	Tazorac" or Avage"	Yes
Retinols	Promote growth of new epithelium; promotes new collagen	Helps remove fine lines and pigment; improves the look of the skin	When used with hydro-quinone	EpiQuin"	Yes
Hydroquinone	Removes pigment	Lightens brown spots	Yes	Claripel", EpiQuin", Glyquin"	Yes
Alpha-hydroxy acids (AHAs); glycolic acid	Exfoliation; collagen production	Improve fine lines	Yes	Glyquin"	Yes

Product	Action	Effect	Proven to work	Brand names	Dr Seckel recommends
Vitamin C ester (L-ascorbic acid)	Antioxidant free-radical scavenger; promotes collagen production; protection from sun	Improves fine lines and skin texture	Yes	Vitamin C Serum˜	Yes
Vitamin E	Antioxidant and sun protection, especially in combination with vitamin C	Prevents ageing changes caused by sun	No	Glyquin˜	Yes
Alpha-lipoic acid (ALA)	Antioxidant	Improves skin texture	No		No
Coenzyme Q10; ubiquinone	Antioxidant	Unknown	No		No
Idebenone		Unknown	No	Prevage˜	No
Polyenyl-phosphatidyl choline (PPC)	Antioxidant; moisturiser	Improves skin texture	No		No
Dimethyl-aminoethanol (DMAE)	Stimulates facial muscle contraction	'Face-lift in a jar'	No		No
Acetyl hexapeptide-3	Relaxes facial muscles	'Better than Botox˜'	No	Avotox˜, StriVectin-SD˜, Creme de Vie˜, Hydroderm˜	No
Palmitoyl pentapeptide	Stimulates collagen and elastin production	Gentle retinol effects	No		No
Hyaluronic acid (HA)	Moisturising skin component	Moisturiser; softens skin	No		No

Personally, all my patients are using a topical cream or solution containing at least one of the following components, which have been scientifically proven to work:

❦ Retin-A™ or Tazarotine™,

❦ alpha-hydroxy acids – glycolic acid,

❦ vitamin C ester L-ascorbic acid),

❦ vitamin E.

Topical creams and solutions are only one very small skirmish in the facial anti-ageing battle, however. Their appeal is that they are so easy to use, but you know all too well by this stage of your life that nothing really good comes easily! Read on.

References
1. Murphy, R. Cosmaceuticals: can they support the claims? *Skin & Ageing* 9:1, 2001.
2. Nyirady, J., Bergfeld, W., Ellis, C. et al. Tretinoin cream 0.02 per cent for the treatment of photo-damaged facial skin: a review of 2 double-blind clinical studies. *Cutis.* 68:135, 2001.
3. Draelos, D. Evaluating vitamin formulations. *J. Aesth. Dermatol. and Cos. Surg.* 1:121, 1999.
4. Bernstein, E.F., Lee, J., Brown, D.B. et al. Glycolic acid treatment increases Type I collagen mRNA and hyaluronic acid content of human skin. *Dermatol. Surg.* 27:5, 2001.
5. Kurtzwell, P. Alpha hydroxyl acids for skincare – smooth sailing or rough seas? *FDA Consumer Magazine* March/April:298, 1999.
6. Perricone, N. *The Perricone Prescription*, 1st edn. New York: Harper Collins, 2002, p. 113.
7. Greul, A.K., Grundmann, J.U., Heinrich, F. et al. Photoprotection of UV-irradiated human skin: an antioxidative combination of vitamins E and C, carotenoids, selenium and proanthocyanidins. *Skin Pharmacol. Appl. Skin Physiol.* 15:307, 2002.
8. Lupo, M.P. Antioxidants and vitamins in cosmetics. *Clin. Dermatol.* 19:467, 2001.
9. Perricone, N. *The Wrinkle Cure*, 1st edn. New York: Warner, 2001, pp. 67–80.
10. Beitner, H. Randomised, placebo controlled, double blind study on the efficacy of a cream containing 5 per cent alpha-lipoic acid related to photo-ageing of facial skin. *Br. J. Dermatol.* 149:841, 2003.
11. Navder, K.P. and Baraona, E. Polyenylphosphatidylcholine attenuates alcohol-induced fatty liver and hyperlipemia in rats. *J. Nutr.* 127:1800, 1997.
12. Uhoda, I., Faska, N. and Robert, C. Split-face study on the cutaneous tensile effect of 2-dimethylaminoethanol (Deanol) gel. *Skin Res. Technol.* 8:164, 2002.
13. Casey, D.E. Mood alterations during Deanol therapy. *Psychopharmacology (Berl)* 62:187, 1979.

7 'No down time' facial anti-ageing procedures

The treatments covered in this chapter are my absolute favourite non-surgical therapies for facial rejuvenation. They are perfect for the busy lifestyle we all have, which does not permit us to have 'down time' away from family, work or friends. More importantly, they work! You will see either an immediate result or results in a couple of weeks (Botox™), at most. If the result is not immediately visible, you will feel the difference in your skin very soon after the procedure.

For a person like me (and most of my patients) with a surgical temperament, waiting for months, looking hopefully in the mirror to see minor skin improvements (if we're lucky) from creams and lotions is not an option!

Within this group of therapies are some of the most beneficial, effective, modern treatments in existence today, provided they are performed by someone who is expert in their use. By 'expert' I mean a doctor or a medical professional (nurse, physician assistant (PA) or

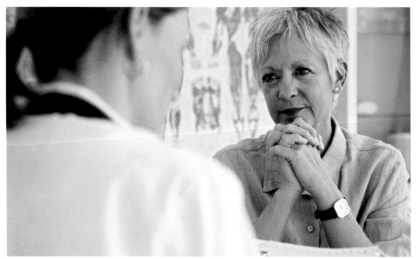

Establish a good relationship with your doctor.

medical aesthetician) who is under the doctor's supervision. Some of the treatments should be done with a supervising doctor present in the facility, and some should only be done by a physician.

The whole idea of doctor supervision is to make certain you are receiving the proper therapy and to guarantee your safety if something goes wrong. Treatments that involve injection, such as fillers, must be done by a physician. If you doubt me, skip ahead and read Chapter 10, 'Don't let "just anyone" touch your face!'

Microdermabrasion – Derma Genesis™

Microdermabrasion is my favourite 'no down time' procedure. In my office, a medical aesthetician performs the procedure under my supervision. The medical aesthetician passes a small tube (which has sand-like particles rushing through it) across the patient's face and places a small opening in the tube on the skin. The skin is gently sucked into the tube, into the stream of rushing particles, which resurface or exfoliate the skin, removing sebum, unblocking pores and removing dead skin cells and superficial pigment.

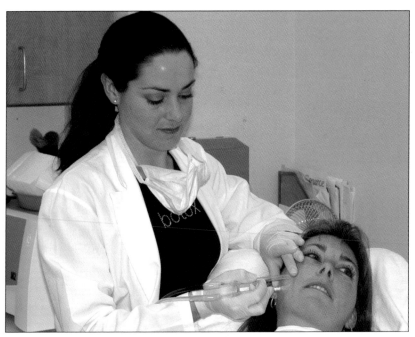

Microdermabrasion is a painless, 'no down time' procedure with wonderful results for your skin.

We use the microdermabrasion machine made by Derma Genesis™, which is capable of a deep effective peel. Having this procedure done in a physician's office has the following benefits.

❦ A doctor is present and can write a prescription for a topical agent that works.

❦ Stronger peel solutions can be used if necessary.

❦ Some people need a **MicroPeel**™ or other treatment not available in a beauty shop. In a physician's office, the appropriate treatment can be determined and offered to you.

❦ In the rare instances in which something goes wrong, the doctor is available immediately.

❦ Certain medical conditions and/or medications require special attention and modification of the procedure.

❦ Prophylactic prescription anti-herpes medication is required for those individuals prone to herpes outbreaks on the face.

❦ Pre-cancerous or cancerous lesions on the face can often be detected at an early stage by a physician.

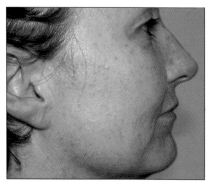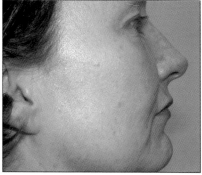

*A patient with hyperpigmentation and Type I ageing changes before (left)
and after (right) a series of microdermabrasion treatments.*

Following microdermabrasion, the skin looks and feels smooth and refreshed. Because dead skin has been removed, topical treatments such as Retin-A™, retinol, alpha-hydroxy acids (AHAs) and vitamin C can more easily penetrate the skin. Skin biopsies have shown that following six microdermabrasion treatments, the epithelium is thicker and healthier looking and there is an increase in superficial dermal collagen. Both are important goals in any anti-ageing treatment.[1] In addition to providing significant microscopic improvement in the skin, microdermabrasion patients report high satisfaction with the treatment in clinical studies.[2, 3] This treatment effectively removes superficial hyperpigmentation when used in conjunction with the appropriate prescription topical agents. The results after a series of treatments over several months are truly remarkable and gratifying.

Microdermabrasion is most effective if used in an overall, multi-step rejuvenation programme involving prescription topical creams and other more invasive procedures, which only can be done in a physician's office.

MicroPeel™

MicroPeel™ is a combination of **dermaplaning** (scraping dead skin off the face) and the subsequent application of a dilute AHA (glycolic acid). This is referred to as 'the lunchtime peel' because pinkness is minimal and you can go back to work after it has been

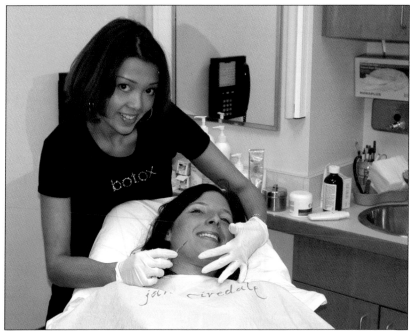

MicroPeel™ is a painless, 'no down time' procedure with wonderful results for your skin.

done. This procedure was developed by Biomedic™ as a useful adjunct to anti-ageing therapies and is suitable for patients who have sensitive skin and cannot tolerate microdermabrasion.

This procedure is only available in physicians' offices, as Biomedic™ does not allow its product to be sold to salons and spas. This is a safety issue, and Biomedic™ is to be congratulated for putting patient safety and ethics ahead of profit.

The benefit to you, the patient, is that in a physician's office you will receive the appropriate procedure and, if needed, a prescription for a topical agent that will enhance the benefit of the MicroPeel™ procedure.

It is also very helpful for acne patients. MicroPeel Plus™ is also available, with added salicylic acid, which makes the peel go a little bit deeper for more effective exfoliation and the stimulation of new collagen growth in the dermis.

Superficial chemical peels

Superficial peels with AHAs of 20–30 per cent or salicylic acid can be applied by medical aestheticians in a doctor's office. These peels provide exfoliation and removal of superficial pigment and can also stimulate new collagen production.

The deeper peels, with a high percentage of AHAs (50–70 per cent), TCA (trichloroacetic acid) peels and phenol peels are considered surgical procedures, to be performed by physicians. These are not minimally invasive. Deeper peels such as these can be very effective, but there is significant down time.

I do not use deep peels because the risks of scarring and **hypopigmentation** (whitening of the treated skin) are too great. Most physicians today prefer laser resurfacing if a deeper peel is needed. Laser resurfacing is a much more controllable, less risky form of facial resurfacing (see Chapter 8). Some doctors obtain beautiful results with the deeper peels and are more experienced than I am in their use. I have seen too many patients who have suffered complications after another doctor has done their peel, and at that point, unfortunately, there is nothing I can do to help them.

MicroLaserPeel™

MicroLaserPeel™ is a new, superficial form of **erbium laser** peel, which is very exciting. Whereas microdermabrasion can remove 5–8

119

microns of skin (1 **micron** is one-thousandth of a millimetre or one-millionth of a metre), an erbium MicroLaserPeel™ can remove 10–20 microns of skin without producing significant down time. The goal is exfoliation and irritation of the dermis to produce new collagen and to enhance the penetration of topical agents such as Retin-A™, retinols, AHAs and vitamin C. Deeper (30–40 microns) MicroLaserPeels™ are more effective, but the skin will be pink for 3–5 days.

The erbium MicroLaserPeel™ is a procedure that is more effective than microdermabrasion because it can remove more tissue and have a more intense effect on the dermal collagen to stimulate new collagen production. Deeper pigmentation can be removed by this technique than by microdermabrasion alone. Although the skin may be pink for a few days, depending on the depth of treatment (see list below), the recovery is not nearly as prolonged as it is with laser resurfacing (see Chapter 9). The results are very gratifying.

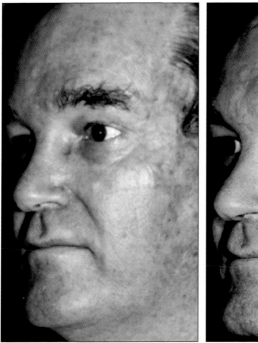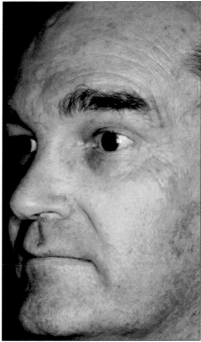

*Before (left) and after (right) a 40-micron MicroLaserPeel™;
the patient's face was pink for 1 week.*

- 10-micron peel: pink for 1–2 days.

- 20-micron peel: pink for 2–3 days.

- 40-micron peel: pink for 5–7 days.

CO_2 Lite™

CO_2 Lite™ is a new feature on the 'gold standard' laser resurfacing machine called the UltraPulse Encore™ made by Lumenis™. The CO_2 Lite™ is a modified, less powerful, carbon-dioxide treatment designed to achieve exfoliation without the prolonged down time of CO_2 laser resurfacing. Recovery times are similar to those for the MicroLaserPeel™ and the treatment takes less time to perform.

Fraxel™

The Fraxel™ procedure is actually an ablative laser procedure (see Chapter 8). Fraxel™, a laser, uses a new approach called **fractional photothermolysis**, thus the name Fraxel™. The laser beam is broken up into tiny beams that are spread apart so that not all areas of the skin are ablated. Rather, tiny 'cells' of skin called microscopic treatment zones (MTZs) are ablated beneath the skin, leaving the surrounding skin intact.

The result is that the skin is inflamed so that new collagen will form, but much of the skin stays in place, so the face is not left raw, as it is after laser resurfacing, and recovery time is shorter.

This is still an ablative laser, the skin does peel afterwards and is red to pink – so I would disagree with statements that this is a 'no down time' procedure, although the down time is less than that with traditional laser resurfacing. However, multiple treatments over a period of 5 weeks are required to get a result. So expect that after each treatment you will be red and have flaking skin for several days.

Fraxel™ is certainly more effective than the 'non-ablative' therapies available today. Just don't plan on going to a social event the evening after having this procedure done.

Photofacial (fotofacial) or photo rejuvenation

These terms are used to market and describe rejuvenation treatments that use intense pulsed light (IPL, see Chapter 8) to rejuvenate the skin. An intense pulsed light beam is flashed on to the face in a series of five to seven treatments over several months.

The main benefit of these treatments is removal of pigment and blood vessels or pink flush from the face. Some patients notice an improvement in skin texture. However, significant wrinkle removal is not seen in many patients. The best result reported is a 20 per cent improvement in wrinkles after 5–7 months.

Botox™

Botox™ is the most revolutionary and effective facial anti-ageing treatment since the advent of laser resurfacing. However, unlike laser resurfacing, there is no down time with the procedure, which, along with the effectiveness of Botox™, accounts for its incredible popularity. The name Botox™ is short for botulinum toxin, a toxin produced by the bacteria *Clostridium botulinum*. It was discovered in 1895 and purified as botulinum toxin A (the type we use today) in 1946. It was first used in the late 1970s to treat torticollis and other severe forms of muscle spasm and was found to be very safe and effective.

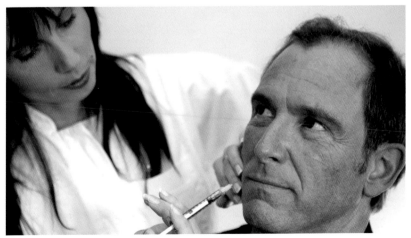

Botox™ works by weakening the muscles of facial expression.

In the 1980s, Doctors Jean and Alastair Carruthers noticed that when they used Botox™ to treat patients with ocular spasm (spasm of the eyelid), the wrinkles or crow's feet around the treated eye disappeared.[4] These results encouraged doctors to use Botox™ to treat the lines of facial expression, frown lines, worry lines, and crow's feet. The cosmetic use of Botox™ was approved by the US Food and Drug Administration (FDA) in April 2002 and, more recently, in the UK.

Botox™ works by weakening the muscles of facial expression. When you contract or tighten one of these muscles, the nerve that connects with it releases a chemical called acetylcholine. The acetylcholine then stimulates the muscle to contract (tighten). Botox™ works by blocking the effect of acetylcholine on the muscle, and causes the muscle to relax and stop pulling on the skin, which results in the wrinkle caused by the muscle pull going away.

Importantly, the muscles of facial expression function to produce an expression on your face. Those that we treat with Botox™ are not involved in chewing or other important functional tasks. If they were, we would not use Botox™ on them. Botox™ also works well on the bunny lines, those little lines at the base of your nose when you squint or wrinkle your nose.

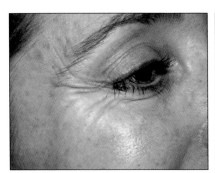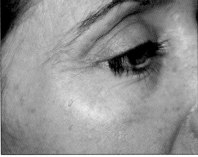

Before (left) and 3 weeks after (right) Botox™ injections for crow's feet; the patient is actively smiling in both photographs.

The part of the eyelid muscle directly beneath the eyelid is important for eye closure and is not treated with Botox™. We treat only the outer part of that muscle, which causes the crow's feet.

Botox™ injections are quick and relatively painless, especially when the area to be injected is iced first and a small 32-gauge needle is used.

Doctors who are expert at the use of Botox™ can also use it to lessen lipstick lines and some of the deep furrows below the lip on the chin. Only small amounts, 2 or 3 IU (International Units), are used in these areas.

Correction of the lines of facial expression is not permanent, so Botox™ injections must be repeated. The initial injection lasts for 3–6 months, but the second injection often lasts 6–9 months. In my experience, the effect of Botox™ on the muscle seems to be cumulative, raising the possibility that after 2–3 years of use, the muscles will have atrophied and may be weak enough to make repeat injections unnecessary. At the present time, however, you should assume that you will continue to need Botox™ injections every 6–9 months for as long as you want the lines to be gone.

It is essential that physicians who inject Botox™ should be experienced in the injection techniques for this drug. Botox™ must be accurately placed within the muscle for it to work; the muscular anatomy of the face is very complex and injections can easily be placed too deeply (below the muscle), or too superficially (in the dermis). In either case, the injection will not work as well and you will be unhappy with the result. It looks so simple, but technique is very important. If Botox™ is placed into the wrong muscle, your eyelid can droop or your smile can become crooked. So ask the right questions when you seek this treatment.

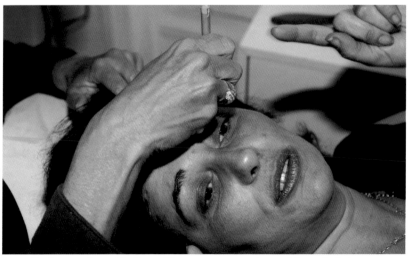

Early results with Botox™ are encouraging, although it is not a cheap treatment.

Adverse reactions that have been reported are headaches (13 per cent), nausea (3 per cent), and flu-like syndrome (2 per cent), but whether they are related to the Botox™ is unknown. Three per cent of patients in initial studies had temporary eyelid droop lasting 3–6 weeks, but in my opinion eyelid droop can be avoided by proper injection technique.

Botox™ injections sting, but the discomfort can be significantly reduced by icing the area prior to injection and diluting the Botox™ with a preservative containing saline (salt water).

Botox™ comes from the manufacturer as a powder, which must be refrigerated. It must be mixed and diluted with saline prior to injection and, once diluted, must be kept refrigerated. The company that makes Botox™ recommends that once diluted and refrigerated, it should be used within 2 weeks, or it will lose much of its effectiveness.

Botox™ is expensive. Treatments are charged by the unit; a typical initial treatment uses 25 units. Fifty units is usually the maximum recommended for one session. In my practice, 50 units could easily treat frown lines, worry lines, crow's feet and bunny lines. Very small amounts (1–3 units) are used around the mouth for lipstick lines, carefully placed to avoid the corner of the mouth, where smile muscles and the muscles used for chewing are present.

We still don't know the long-term effects of Botox™ treatment on the muscles, but it has been in clinical use since 1978 and no adverse long-term effects have been reported. Recent widely publicised stories of complications in Florida were misleading. The individuals involved did not use Botox™, but rather an unapproved solution manufactured in a laboratory. Please re-read the first section of this chapter and Chapter 10 about the importance of finding an accredited, ethical doctor for your facial rejuvenation treatments.

Fillers

As we learned in Chapter 2, facial wrinkles and lines, other than lines of facial expression, are formed when our skin loses collagen, subcutaneous fat and elasticity and becomes lax. One solution is to inject a filler substance such as collagen into the deeper layer of the skin, the dermis, to plump up the depression or wrinkle. There is a wide variety of excellent fillers available today; in fact, so many products, which are so aggressively marketed, that it can be very confusing for you to know which filler, if any, is most suitable for you. You must rely on the knowledge of your physician, and it is therefore important to find a doctor who is knowledgeable about all of the fillers that are available. In my experience, each of the various types of filler has a specific application. The proper filler expertly placed in the appropriate patient produces a pleasing result.

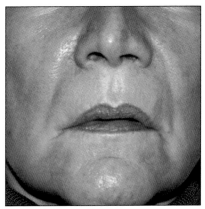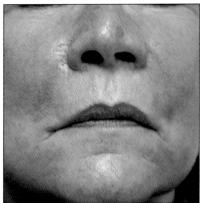

Before (left) and after (right) Radiesse™ injection
into the nasal–labial fold lines.

Fillers are very popular and there are many new exciting types available today. However, there are two things you should keep in mind when considering using a filler.

First, fillers are a camouflage: they make the wrinkle or line less noticeable, but they do nothing to correct the basic problem. The problem that caused the wrinkle in the first place – loss of collagen, elastin and subcutaneous fat and the action of the facial muscles pulling on the skin for many years – is still present and is not corrected by the injection of a filler.

For example, in the case of the nasal–labial fold line (see Chapter 1), we plump the line by injecting filler deep into the dermis underneath it. This plumps the skin and makes the line less noticeable, but it is still present, and still caused by the overhanging, sagging cheek. A more corrective procedure would be to pull the cheek up and tighten it – that would be a face-lift. However, many patients do not want to undergo a surgical procedure, preferring to improve the facial ageing change rather

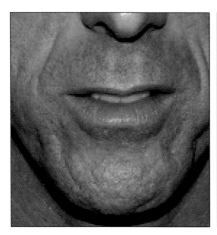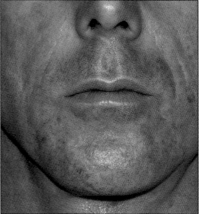

Before (left) and after (right) Restylane™ injection into the nasal–labial fold line, cheek wrinkle and chin creases.

than surgically correct it. For these patients, fillers are an excellent alternative.

Secondly, most fillers are temporary. Since they are foreign protein derived from animal sources (cow, pig, rooster comb), the body recognises them as foreign proteins and degrades and removes them, in some cases after as little as 3 weeks! More permanent fillers are available, but there are risks. Silicone, for example, one of the first fillers used, is permanent, but it is not FDA approved because there is a high risk of complications, called granulomas. These are nasty, permanent bumps in the skin which can open, become infected and drain. So we'll stick with our discussion of safer, FDA-approved filler substances.

Collagen – Zyderm™, Zyderm I™, Zyplast™

Collagen (widely used in the form of Zyplast™) is a commonly used filler. It has been chemically altered to be less **allergenic** (less likely to cause an allergic reaction), and also lasts longer than earlier forms. It is injected into the dermis to plump up the skin and can be used to treat lines, scars and other depressions.

There are two main problems with collagen. The first is that roughly 3 per cent of people are allergic to it, the allergy showing up as a nasty red bump. A simple skin test similar to a tuberculosis (TB) test is done on your arm, and a positive result after 4 weeks means that you are allergic to collagen. Only after 4 weeks and a

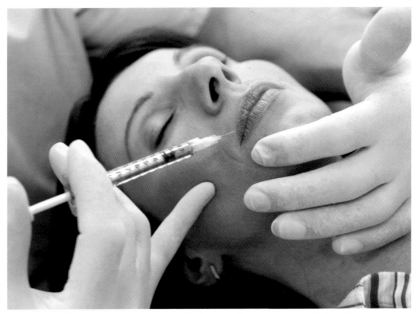

Collagen treatment can help to plump areas of the face.

negative skin test can you receive a collagen injection. The second drawback with collagen is that it does not last very long, usually no longer than 3 months.

However, it has many advantages. Collagen products contain an anaesthetic, which makes injection less painful. It is also less expensive per cm³ than the newer fillers. I like the fact that I have much more volume when using Zyplast™ and can easily treat several areas of the face.

Hyaluronic acid – Restylane™, Perlane™, Hylaform™

Do not confuse injectable hyaluronic acid (HA), which is a filler, with the HA creams discussed in the last chapter; the creams are just moisturisers. Also, HA the filler is temporary and is used for its plumping action on the skin. Injectable HA has no magical anti-ageing effects on your skin.

HA is a newer filler with several advantages over collagen. First, allergy to HA is not an issue, so skin testing is not required. Early studies indicate that HA may last longer than collagen, possibly up to 6–8 months – another distinct advantage.

HA is marketed as Restylane™, Restylane Fine Lines™, Perlane™

and Hylaform™. All these products contain HA; it's just the size of the HA particles that varies. Restylane Fine Lines™ has the smallest particle size and is placed high in the superficial dermis to treat fine lines. Restylane™ has larger particles and is placed in the mid-dermis to treat moderately deep nasal–labial fold lines and in lip rejuvenation to plump up the lip. Perlane™ has the largest particle and is placed in the deep dermis or subcutaneous fat to correct deep folds and to do facial contouring in patients with sunken cheeks.

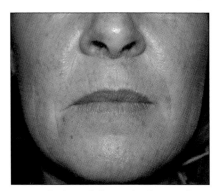 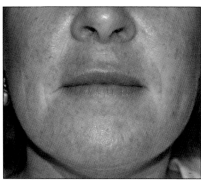

Lips before (left) and after (right) a Restylane™ injection; note the lip is fuller and the lipstick lines are less noticeable after the filler injection.

Unlike collagen, HA does not contain an anaesthetic. Therefore I use a topical anaesthetic to numb the skin first, or nerve blocks (like the dentist), although that is rarely necessary. The Restylane™ fillers consist of HA that has been biologically engineered from bacteria. It is a mucopolysaccharide, not a protein like collagen, so is less likely to produce an allergic reaction. Hylaform™ is made from rooster comb.

One syringe (about 1 cm³ – approximately a third of the volume of a syringe of Zyplast™) of HA can usually treat the lips and mild or superficial nasal–labial fold lines. Deeper nasal–labial fold lines require two syringes. It's high tech, but it's expensive.

'Permanent' or long-lasting fillers – Radiesse™, Artefill™ and Sculptra™

Radiesse™, Artefill™ and Sculptra™ are new fillers that are marketed as long-lasting or permanent. *They are not permanent!* These ingeniously conceived, high-tech fillers are also injected with a needle. Once injected, they stimulate your body to form your own tissue around the filler, producing a long-lasting result.

Radiesse™ is an injectable implant, scientifically designed to provide biocompatibility, durability, efficacy and ease of use in soft-tissue augmentation. The primary compound used in Radiesse™ is pure, synthetic calcium hydroxylapatite (CaHA) particles composed of calcium and phosphate ions. Because these occur naturally in the body, they are inherently biocompatible and are by nature non-irritant to the body. Radiesse™ has been used for decades as an implant material in plastic and reconstructive surgery, orthopaedics, otology, otolaryngology, neurosurgery, dentistry, maxillofacial surgery and urology.

Artefill™ uses polymethyl methacrylate (PMMA) spheres suspended in collagen. Over a 3-month period after an injection, your own collagen grows in around the spheres, resulting in a 'permanent' fill.

Sculptra™ is the latest filler, made of poly-L-lactic acid, a substance that has been used for many years as suture material. Sculptra™ is quite different from Radiesse™ and Artefill™ in that it comes in a powder form, which must be diluted with saline and lidocaine, an anaesthetic. Also, the treatments must be repeated once or twice before the final fill is achieved. Once it is in place, it is long lasting, but it is more complicated to use than Radiesse™ and Artefill™.

The main problem with long-lasting or permanent fillers is that we don't know what the long-term (10–15 years) effect is going to be. They have been used for the past 2–5 years, especially in Europe, and have been successful and safe enough to gain FDA approval in the USA. The honest answer is that we don't know if there are going to be long-term negative effects.

Permanent and long-lasting fillers must be injected into the mid-dermis or deeper. Superficial injection can produce granulomas, and they are not FDA approved for use in the lips because of this risk.

I always insist that patients try the non-permanent fillers, like collagen or HA, first, to see if they like the effect. If a patient is happy with temporary fillers and is fully aware of the uncertainty and the potential long-term risks of more permanent fillers, I will then consider using one. Long-term fillers are the most expensive, although prices are coming down as a result of competition from the HA fillers.

I do like the way Radiesse™ fills the nasal–labial fold line.

The ultimate filler – your own fat

Your own fat can be harvested (removed) from an area of your body that doesn't need it (such as your hips) and injected back into your face to treat nasal–labial fold lines, puff up the lips and fill the tear trough deformity. However, fat injection around the eyes for the tear trough deformity is very tricky, and personally I prefer **blepharoplasty** with muscle repositioning (see Chapter 9). Fat from your own body has the advantage of not being a foreign substance, so you don't need to worry about an allergic reaction.

Fat transplantation is a somewhat complex technique. Only about 35–50 per cent of transplanted fat cells survive the process. Therefore most surgeons attempt to over-correct – in other words, they transplant 35–50 per cent more fat than needed for the desired correction, allowing for shrinkage due to loss of the fat cells that don't survive the transplantation process.

Why don't we use this technique more often? Because it is surgery, which requires skill and training, and there is a 2–3-week recovery period, during which you will be very swollen and bruised. Thus it is not a 'no down time' technique. However, if you don't want to bother with repeated filler injections, you don't mind the recovery period and you can find a surgeon skilled in this technique, fat transplantation can be a very beneficial treatment.

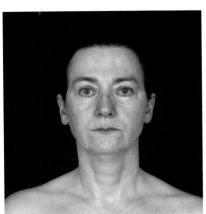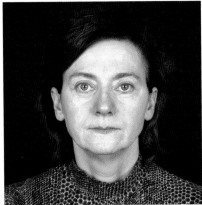

Before (left) and after (right) a fat transplantation technique.

Caution about fillers

The results or benefits you will see after the injection of any filler, whether it's collagen, Restylane™, Radiesse™ or fat, are only as good as the skill of the person who injects these substances into your face. The injection of a filler requires skill, expertise, and experience. It looks so simple on the videotapes that the filler companies give to doctors as marketing tools. It is not simple. I have been doing it for 23 years and I still don't do it perfectly every time. An inexperienced physician can easily push all the filler into the subcutaneous fat, which will have no effect on the wrinkle. Alternatively, it can be placed too superficially, just under the skin or epithelium, where it can cause a noticeable bump or, worse, a granuloma.

This is not something you want the occasional user to do to your face! Ask your doctor the right questions – How often does he or she do this? Is he/she experienced? – and ask other people how satisfied they were with the experience they had with the same doctor. The thought of a nurse or non-physician administering a filler injection simply horrifies me!

The Thread Lift™, Feather Lift™, Russian Lift™ or Contour Lift™

The terms Thread Lift™, Feather Lift™, Russian Lift™ and Contour Lift™ are used to describe a technique for lifting the facial skin using small 'threads' that are placed beneath it, attached to its underside, and then pulled upwards to tighten it.

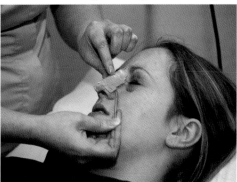

Lifting the facial skin uses small threads beneath the skin.

The threads are placed beneath the skin using a needle, which is passed through the skin at a point low in the cheek, under the cheek skin up to a point higher on the face, and then back out through the skin. The thread has small barbs sticking out, which attach to the under-surface of the skin and pull up on it as the thread is tightened from above.

Although these procedures are being marketed as non-surgical face-lifts, 'no down time' face-lifts, lunch-time face-lifts, and other such terms, you must understand that these are surgical procedures. In fact they are surgical implant procedures, and complications can and do occur.

Before considering one of these procedures you need to be aware of several potential problems:

❦ bruising and down time,

❦ infection,

❦ extrusion – that is, the thread pushes out onto the surface of the skin,

❦ injury to the facial nerve – this can paralyse your face,

❦ 'divits', or visible dents or depressions, in your face,

❦ scarring,

❦ failure to lift the face,

❦ excess skin bulge above the exit point of the needle and thread.

Bruising and down time

Injecting a local anaesthetic (required for these procedures) and passing a needle and thread beneath the skin damage blood vessels and cause bleeding. Bleeding under the skin causes bruising, and you will have bruising following this procedure. Some people can go to work with bruises and swelling on their faces, but most people don't want to. If you have one of these procedures, be prepared for swelling and bruises that can last up to 10 days, sometimes 2 weeks.

Infection

Any time you enter the skin with a needle or other foreign object, bacteria can be pushed into the skin and cause infection. Good surgical technique, scrubbing with an antiseptic solution and using sterile techniques and antibiotics help, but infections can occur despite these precautions.

Placing an implant, such as a thread, under the skin introduces a 'foreign body' and greatly increases the chances of an infection.

Extrusion

Our bodies recognise and try to reject or push out foreign material. A splinter is a good example: notice how the area around the splinter becomes infected and the pus eventually pushes the splinter out. When the body rejects or pushes implanted material out it is called an extrusion.

Although medical devices such as breast implants and the 'threads' can be implanted safely, the material must be perfectly sterile and placed with meticulous, sterile surgical technique. In addition, the body tissue around the implant must be healthy, and generally the deeper the implant is placed in the body, the better the chance that it will not be rejected.

Since the threads are placed close to the surface of the skin, the chances of infection, rejection and extrusion are greater than for implants placed deeper in the body.

Injury to the facial nerve

This is the most dreaded and debilitating of all complications of any facial surgery, including a face-lift. Damage to a facial nerve branch is often permanent and causes paralysis or sagging of the face, inability to smile or raise the forehead, and can cause difficulty closing the eyelids.

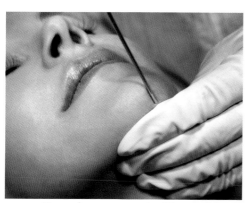

Procedures are not without risk, so you should always consult experienced professionals.

Accredited plastic surgeons spend many years learning how not to injure these nerves during face-lift surgery and understand and recognise the locations of these nerves so that they are avoided and not injured.

The Thread Lift™ is a blind procedure, meaning that the needle and thread are passed beneath the skin without the surgeon being able to see the structures under the skin through which the needle is passing. If the needle is passed a little too deep or through an area where the facial nerve is close to the skin, the nerve can be injured and facial paralysis can result.

'Divits', or visible dents or depressions, in your face

One problem that surgeons can have with the Thread Lift™ is that on occasion the barbed thread catches hold of the underside of the skin tightly in one location on the face. When this happens, the upward pull on the cheek is exerted entirely at that one spot. The cheek is 'hooked' from underneath at that spot and creates a dimple or depression on the skin, resulting in an unsightly deformity.

Scarring

When you break or enter the skin, whether with a scalpel or a needle, it always forms a scar. Of course, a needle puncture creates a smaller scar than a scalpel. However, if the needle – a large one in the case of the Thread Lift™ – passes through the skin, it will always leave a mark.

If the needle needs to be passed through the skin several times to find the right position, and at the exit point where the thread is tightened and tied, a scar is likely to be larger.

If the thread becomes infected or a 'divit' or depression forms, the thread will need to be removed surgically, and a larger scar will result.

Failure to lift the face

Threads can fail and the face can drop.

Excess skin bulge above the exit point of the needle and thread

Take your hands, place them on your cheeks and push your facial skin up to tighten it and make your face look younger. Do you notice the excess skin bulging above your hands high up on your face and around your ears? This is what you will see if you have a face-lift and the surgeon does not remove or cut away the excess facial skin.

This is the biggest limitation and drawback to the Thread Lift™. Although with proper surgical technique the threads can be used to pull the cheek up, if you don't do surgery to remove the excess skin, you will be left with an unsightly bulge. Most websites recommending this procedure say it is only for younger patients, who don't have much excess skin. I would guess that these same people don't need a face-lift anyway.

The Lifestyle Lift™ and the Weekend Lift™

The Lifestyle Lift™ and the Weekend Lift™ are modifications of a full face-lift designed to be less extensive surgical procedures with less down time and a more rapid recovery. In my opinion, they are

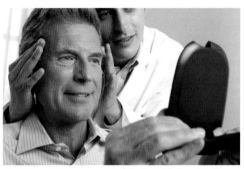

A 'non-surgical' face-lift is still a surgical procedure.

appropriate for younger patients with less excess facial skin who do not require a standard full face-lift.

BE CAUTIOUS! No matter what these operations are called, they are surgical procedures. Surgery can cause bruising and swelling and many people cannot have a surgical procedure on Friday and return to work on Monday. Some people will

have bruising and swelling that can take up to 2 weeks to resolve. Also, as with any surgery, its success will depend on the skill of the surgeon performing it, and not all surgeons are equally skilled or experienced. Personally, I would not call these surgical procedures 'no down time' procedures.

The non-surgical face-lift

The term 'non-surgical face-lift' is advertised widely on the Internet and elsewhere to promote a new skin-tightening procedure that uses radiofrequency waves (Thermage™) or infrared waves (Titan™) to heat the deep layers of the skin and tighten it. These procedures are discussed in detail in Chapter 8. They can produce skin tightening, but they are not face-lifts and do not achieve the same result as a face-lift. They are 'no down time' procedures.

References
1. Rubin, M. and Greenbaum, S.S. Histologic effects of aluminum oxide microabrasion on facial skin. *J. Aesth. Dermatol. Cos. Surg.* 1:237, 2000.
2. Shim, E.K., Barnette, D., Hughes, K. et al. Microdermabrasion: a clinical and histopathologic study. *Dermatol. Surg.* 27:534, 2001.
3. Tan, M., Spencer, J.M. and Pires, L.M. The evaluation of aluminum oxide crystal microdermabrasion for photo-damage. *Dermatol. Surg.* 27:943, 2001.
4. Brown, L.H. and Brancaccio, R.R. Injecting Botox: tips from a master. *Skin & Ageing* 10:38, 2002.

8 High-tech facial rejuvenation: non-ablative therapies

Hold on to your wallets. When you move up from vitamins, meditation, sun block, microdermabrasion, and Retin-A™, you are going to start spending some serious cash. Before you do, let me educate you as to the *truth* about these new and very tempting therapies.

One major problem you have is that the companies that make these machines have spent millions of dollars not only developing and making them but also marketing them. Before the doctors are sure that they work as promised, the companies have already advertised them in glamour magazines and have had testimonials on TV talk shows. The result is that you show up in the doctor's office

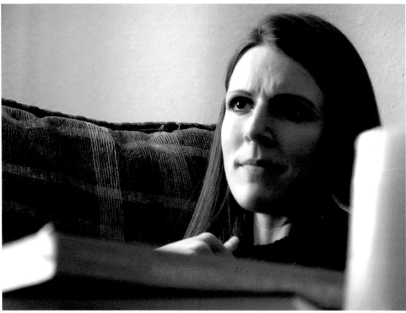

You need to know the full facts in order to make an informed decision.

demanding the treatment and the doctor is backed into a corner – either buy the machine or lose you as a patient. It is a very unhealthy situation for you and the doctor. I urge you to study this chapter carefully.

I will explain to you how these machines work, what they can do for you, what they cannot do for you and, more importantly, how they can hurt you if they are not used correctly. Then you will be empowered to make a good choice.

Some of these machines can do wonderful and remarkable things to reverse ageing changes in your face when used by qualified physicians who are up to date in their knowledge about the various modalities and machines. But you need to be able to wade through the hyperbole and find what you need, and find the appropriate doctor to advise you. There's more on finding the right doctor in Chapter 10, 'Don't let "just anyone" touch your face!'.

What are high-tech non-ablative therapies?

To ablate, as used here, means to remove surgically. Non-ablative, as used in this chapter to describe laser, IPL (intense pulsed light), radiofrequency, infrared light and LED (light-emitting diode) therapies, means that these machines do their work on your skin to remove pigment and blood vessels and stimulate new collagen production *without surgically removing or damaging the top layer (epithelium) of your skin*. The benefits, of course, are that if the skin is not ablated, you will not have the long recovery time associated with ablative laser resurfacing and there will be less risk of scarring.

This is a very sophisticated, highly technical process. These therapies are called non-ablative to distinguish them from the ablative procedure of laser resurfacing, which is done with the more powerful CO_2 and erbium lasers, both of which are discussed in Chapter 9 under plastic surgical procedures. Do not be misled. The machines that are used for non-ablative therapies are powerful enough to cause ablation (removal) of your skin if they are not used properly by someone who is an expert and skilled in their use. In my practice, trained nurses under my supervision do some of these therapies.

Notice, I said 'under my supervision', which means I am present on site at the time most treatments are done. I know that in many states it is legal for some of these therapies to be done at a spa or laser centre by a nurse or technician when the 'medical director', the doctor, is not on site. In my opinion, this is far too dangerous for many of the high-tech therapies. I have seen some terrible complications following supposedly non-ablative laser procedures done by non-medically trained personnel and medical doctors.

Non-ablative facial rejuvenation procedures, when done for the right indication by a qualified person in a doctor's office, are effective and safe and eliminate much of the down time associated with traditional ablative procedures done in the past.

Non-ablative laser and IPL facial rejuvenation

Be very careful here. These services are marketed to you as facial rejuvenation. That can be misleading. All reputable doctors agree that these techniques do a great job removing Type I facial ageing changes such as brown spots and telangiectasias, but most will tell you that these procedures do not remove wrinkles and tighten loose skin, the Type II facial ageing changes. So do not be misled. Non-ablative laser and IPL therapy is very effective for:

* removal of brown spots (pigment),

* removal of telangiectasias (blood vessels around the nose, and on the cheeks and chin).

What about wrinkle removal?

While effective and safe non-ablative therapies have been available to treat brown spots, telangiectasias, hair and tattoos for several years, the technology for wrinkle removal is still new and not nearly as effective and reliable as the other therapies. While some non-ablative laser treatments can stimulate new collagen production and improve skin texture and wrinkles, the results are seen only after repeated treatments, and after 5–7 months.

I want to help you understand how these therapies are supposed to work and what they can and cannot do for you.

How do non-ablative laser and IPL work?

Remember that I told you in Chapter 5 that the ultimate goal of all facial rejuvenation treatments is to remove pigment (brown spots) and telangiectasias (blood vessels) and to restore the old, damaged collagen and elastin that have caused the skin to lose its elasticity and wrinkle. In previous chapters we have discussed how topical agents, exfoliation, Botox™ and fillers are used to attempt to correct these ageing changes. Lasers and IPL attempt to correct ageing changes in a very different, high-tech way.

A phenomenal characteristic of lasers and IPL is that these machines can be manufactured to produce a very powerful beam of light that will only attack or destroy a specifically coloured target. This phenomenon is called **target-specific photothermolysis**. Photothermolysis is the use of light to heat and destroy a tissue such as pigment, a blood vessel, a cell, or collagen and elastin in the skin. The key phrase here is target specific. Unlike a shotgun, bomb or other high-powered form of energy, which destroys everything it hits, a laser or IPL can be tuned or controlled to damage only a tiny target of a specific colour and not injure anything else in the surrounding area. For example, if you want to remove pigment, use a laser or IPL light beam tuned to target only brown pigment. If you want to remove telangiectasias, use a laser or IPL tuned to target only the red colour of the blood inside a blood vessel.

This is possible because a laser or IPL beam is a light beam, an incredibly powerful, high-energy light beam (so powerful that a message can be sent to outer space on the back of a laser beam), which consists of only one colour. The type of gas in the laser tube that is made to generate the laser beam, or the colour of a lens in the IPL machine, determines the colour of the light beam that comes out of the machine. This characteristic allows us to target the light beam to one specifically coloured target – a red blood vessel, or a brown spot, or a blue tattoo.

Once the appropriately coloured light beam reaches the target, the high energy of the light beam (laser beam or IPL light beam), which is very hot, is absorbed by the specifically coloured target. It heats the target and then ruptures or kills it, but does not damage the overlying skin. Thus if you want to remove a brown spot from the skin, you use a laser tuned to be absorbed by brown pigment (Figure 8.1). The skin is cooled as the laser passes through the epidermis into the pigment, which is broken up by the heat from

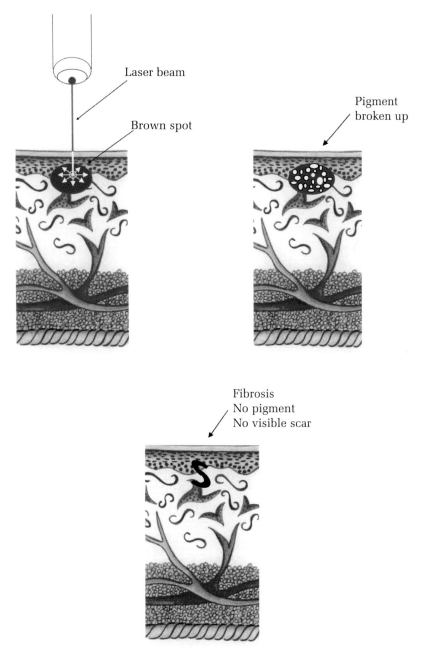

Figure 8.1 A laser beam attacks a brown spot (top left); pigment is broken up (top right); pigment is gone and, after healing, there is no visible scar (bottom).

the laser. Since the epidermis is not injured, there is no scar left behind. So, if you want to destroy something blue in the skin (a tattoo), you shine a powerful laser or IPL light beam tuned only to target blue. The laser will pass through the non-blue skin and be absorbed by, and thus destroy, the blue tattoo pigment. The first clinically useful practical application of the concept of target-specific photothermolysis was in the skin – first for tattoo removal, then for blood vessel and brown spot removal, and then for hair removal.

Non-ablative wrinkle removal

Scientists have been trying for years to perfect this technique to target age-damaged collagen and elastin in the dermis (the deep layer of the skin) without damaging the epidermis (top layer) as the beam passes through on its way to the dermis. If this can be accomplished, the damage to the collagen and elastin caused by the laser or IPL beam results in inflammation, which leads to **fibrosis**. Fibrosis is the production of new collagen in the wounded area by fibroblasts, the collagen-producing cells that come into the dermis after inflammation. Yes, it is a scar, but a controlled scar.

The theory is that if we can cause fibrosis in the dermis without injuring the overlying epidermis, the new collagen should restore elasticity, plump and tighten the skin and remove wrinkles.

We are close, but the technique for wrinkle removal is not as effective as it is for the removal of tattoos, blood vessels, brown spots and hair. Although this concept is theoretically possible, and the newer technology can produce microscopic new collagen regeneration, so far new collagen has been formed only in tiny, barely noticeable amounts. The best results require multiple treatments over months.

More importantly, even though we call these therapies non-ablative, there is some risk of injury. As the laser beam passes through the outer layer of the skin, some of the heat energy heats it, even though the outer skin is not the target, and, potentially, the skin could be burned.

To avoid blistering the outer skin, most lasers and IPL machines used for non-ablative therapies have some sort of device to cool the skin during the treatment so that the hot laser or light beam does not heat and burn (blister) the skin on its way through the epidermis to the dermis. However, all of these machines have the power to burn the skin and create scarring if they are not used properly or if their skin-cooling systems fail. It has happened; I have seen it with my own eyes. One exception is Laser Genesis˝, which requires no skin contact and has shown good results.

If these machines do not remove wrinkles, why in blazes did I drag you through this tedious theoretical discussion? Because soon, probably before I finish my next book, these non-ablative therapies will be improved to a point at which they will work very well.

I want you to understand how they work so you can ask the right questions and pick the right laser. Check my website (www.saveyourface.com) occasionally and I will keep you updated. You will be the first to know when I know, I promise!

The particular name or brand of the laser or IPL is less important than the expertise of the doctor you choose, so see Chapter 10 and learn how to choose the right doctor and then trust him or her to know which laser or IPL is the best one for your treatment.

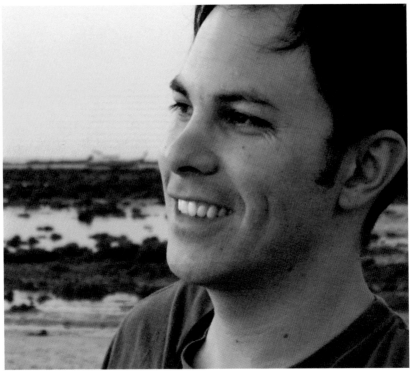

I'll keep you updated on the latest developments in facial rejuvenation.

Infrared light (Titan™), radiofrequency (Thermage™) and FACES™: non-ablative skin tightening – the 'non-surgical face-lift'

The latest generation of infrared light and radiofrequency machines – Titan™, Thermage™ and FACES™ – work very differently from lasers and IPL. Their potential usefulness is based on the fact that when heated to 63 degrees centigrade, collagen shortens or tightens and 'remodels' into a shorter or tighter form. When the collagen in the dermis of the skin treated by these machines is tightened, the skin is tightened. These machines produce 'controlled' deeper heating over a larger area than the intense focused heating produced by a laser. They also use a very sophisticated cooling system to protect the overlying epidermis as the radiofrequency or infrared light energy is passed through the epidermis (Figure 8.2).

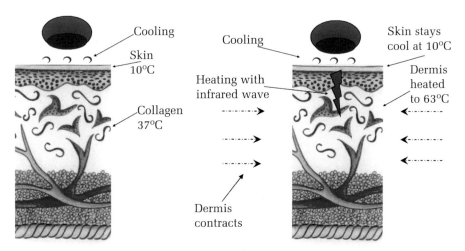

Figure 8.2a In the cooling phase, the skin is cooled prior to passing infrared or radiofrequency energy through the epidermis to heat the dermis.

Figure 8.2b In the cooling and heating phase, the skin is cooled and energy is passed simultaneously into the dermis to heat the collagen in the dermis to 63 °C.

The photographs of patients treated so far with the Titan™ and Thermage™ devices have been impressive. The manufacturers report on average a 30 per cent tightening of the skin.

It takes at least three to five treatments, scheduled several weeks apart, to obtain a result. Although some patients see a result immediately, the final result will usually not be apparent for 3–5 months, the time it takes for the collagen to remodel. This requires patience on the part of the patient, but this new therapy may be a good alternative for those not wanting surgery. The cost of these treatments is determined by the size and difficulty of the area being treated.

One drawback of this exciting non-ablative therapy is that it is a slow, tedious process, often taking an hour to do an entire face. The newer FACES™ treatments are much faster and less painful. Trained nurses and physicians' assistants under the supervision of the doctor can also do the actual treatment.

Complications have been reported with Thermage™, most noticeably depressions or irregularity in the skin of the cheek and the side of the forehead, near the temple. Accordingly, current guidelines recommend not treating those two areas. I do not see that as much of a problem. The areas we can treat – the jowls, neck, turkey wattle, chin, mouth, nasal–labial fold line and forehead – are the areas where ageing changes are most profound.

Titan™ and FACES™ are newer and, to date, I have not heard of complications with these machines.

Not all patients respond to these therapies. I assure you that within a year or so, we will know how to predict more accurately who will and who will not get a good result, how to avoid complications, and how to do a more effective treatment. I suggest you wait a few months and, in the meantime, use the proven therapies outlined in this book. You will make progress in your anti-ageing battle and, who knows, the preparatory work you do may enhance the result you obtain from a high-tech skin-tightening procedure in the future. Also, by next year, there may well be a newer, more effective non-ablative therapy. In fact, I can almost guarantee it. I will keep you posted on my website, www.saveyourface.com.

LED (GentleWaves™)

LED stands for light-emitting diode. LEDs are those little red lights that blink when you press the remote control for your TV set. You also see them on your microwave and other appliances. Why would anyone think of using them to treat facial ageing?

According to the people who sell GentleWaves™, a scientist in the US space programme was studying LEDs because, I assume, our astronauts are frequently exposed to a lot of them during space flight. Scientists discovered that when fibroblasts growing in culture in a laboratory were exposed to LEDs they made more collagen than when they were not. If LEDs can stimulate collagen production by fibroblasts in the laboratory, then they might be able to do the same thing in human skin. Right? Studies reveal some evidence to suggest that this concept may be correct.

While clinical results were not as dramatic as they were with other non-ablative therapies, the LED treatments are very simple, safe, painless and brief. Five seconds is all a treatment requires, and the patient feels nothing. The skin does not tighten and wrinkles do not disappear. However, Type I ageing skin changes – brown spots, pigment, telangiectasias, rosacea – and skin texture are all reported to be improved after 5 weeks of one 5-second treatment per week. The improvement is not as dramatic as it is with the laser and IPL.

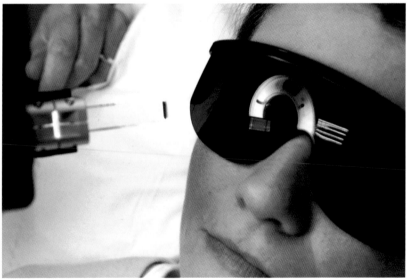

LED treatment can stimulate collagen formation.

However, this treatment is new, and long-term controlled studies of its effectiveness have not been completed, so the jury is still out on this therapy. But preliminary results are encouraging, especially considering the simple, safe, painless and quick nature of the treatment. It also costs about the same as a 'face-lift in a jar' or a 'better than Botox™' and is definitely quicker. You will be examined by a physician before the treatment, who should also prescribe a retinoid or other proven effective skin preparation. When I know more about LEDs and their effectiveness, I will alert you on my website, www.saveyourface.com.

After this lengthy technical discussion, what can non-ablative therapies do for you today (Table 8.1)? A great deal!

❀ They can effectively and quickly correct Type I facial ageing changes, such as brown spots, telangiectasias and rosacea, and remove unwanted hair without the scarring associated with traditional surgical methods of removal.

❀ With multiple treatments, over a period of several months, skin texture and minor wrinkling can be improved.

❀ They can tighten the skin (of some of you) by about 30 per cent, especially in very thin individuals with very little subcutaneous fat.

Table 8.1 What non-ablative therapies can and cannot do

Ageing change	Non-ablative lasers	IPL	LED	FACES™, Titan™, Thermage™
Remove pigment	Yes	Yes	Slowly	No
Remove blood vessels	Yes	Yes	Slowly	No
Improve skin texture	Slowly	Slowly	Slowly	No
Remove fine wrinkles	Slowly	Slowly	No	No
Tighten skin	No	No	No	Yes

IPL = intense pulsed light; LED = light-emitting diode.

These are dramatic and exciting new weapons in the anti-ageing arsenal. Yes, they are more expensive than the 'face-lift in a jar' and 'better than Botox™', but these therapies actually work, and in the long run will probably save you money.

More importantly, when these therapies are combined with the 'no down time' treatments discussed in Chapter 7 and the prescription skin creams listed in Chapter 6, you will definitely see visible, gratifying reversal of Type I facial ageing changes when you look in the mirror! If you also make the dietary, supplement and lifestyle changes discussed in Chapter 4, you will amplify these exciting results, you will feel much better, and you will probably live longer! Who could ask for more?

9 *What can plastic surgery do for you?*

Modern, properly executed plastic surgery operations can dramatically restore the aged human face to a much younger appearance. Plastic surgery can often make a face look 20 or 30 years younger than the person's chronological age.

I have placed my discussion of plastic surgery near the end of this book, which is where it should be. All surgeons are taught to practise under the principle that surgery is the last option. Surgery is only to be considered when:

❦ all non-surgical medical therapies have failed,

❦ no medical therapies exist that can produce as effective a result or cure as surgery.

In this book, I have tried to educate you about most of the newer non-surgical treatments. Having done so, I now feel free to tell you about the surgical options. Cosmetic plastic surgery is elective, so the decision to have surgery must ultimately be reached by you. The decision about when the more minor non-surgical options can be considered to have failed is often a subjective one and requires sound, honest advice from your plastic surgeon.

Plastic surgery as a specialty has undergone a revolutionary and exciting transformation during my

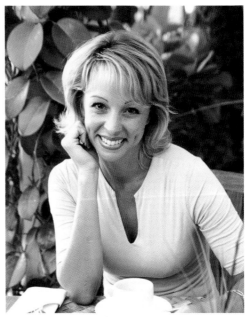

Treatments for facial ageing are safer and more effective than ever.

25 years in this field. Research, education and continued improvement and refinement of anti-ageing techniques are rigorously pursued by plastic surgery societies and all reputable plastic surgeons. The result is that, at the time of writing, the surgical techniques available for the reversal of facial ageing are better, more effective and safer than I would have believed possible when I was in training more than 27 years ago. So if you are contemplating plastic surgery, let me assure you that the surgical procedures available to you are as technologically advanced and exciting as the antioxidant, holistic and non-ablative therapies discussed earlier in this book.

Since the purpose of this book is to inform you about the available options to rejuvenate your face (not to provide a textbook to teach you how to perform plastic surgery), I will only briefly and generally discuss the more common facial rejuvenation procedures. These operations can truly rejuvenate your face and can give you a remarkable, lasting and beautiful result if your expectations as a patient are realistic and if the procedure is performed by a competent plastic surgeon.

You notice I said 'patient'. You are a 'client' when you buy lipstick or skinceuticals. The minute a doctor touches you, you are a 'patient'. Don't forget it and always insist on it, please!

Laser resurfacing

Laser resurfacing of the face is one of the most revolutionary new procedures for reversing facial ageing to have been developed in the past 25 years. The ablative CO_2 and erbium lasers can remove wrinkles, tighten skin and make your face look decades younger. But don't be fooled: laser resurfacing is surgery. Laser resurfacing creates a wound on your face. When a wound is created, you have had surgery.

In Chapter 2, you learned how ageing damage to the epithelium and collagen of your facial skin results in wrinkles and other ageing changes. I told you that all anti-ageing therapies attempt to make your skin new by stimulating the production of new epithelial cells and collagen. That is exactly what laser resurfacing does, all at once and very aggressively.

The laser strips off the old epithelium and partially removes and injures the old, damaged collagen and elastin in the dermis. As a result of this injury, macrophages migrate from the blood into the skin, remove the damaged tissue and convert to fibroblasts to create new collagen. New epithelial cells grow over the face and form a new, young-looking epidermis. After the face has fully healed, the facial skin is tighter, fresher looking and wrinkle free.

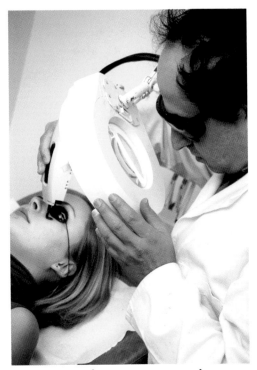

The reason laser resurfacing has been such a revolutionary and rapidly accepted new procedure in plastic surgery is that this technique enabled us to correct facial-ageing changes that a face-lift could not correct. While a face-lift could correct jowling and tighten loose skin, patients were often disappointed by the fact that their facial skin still had fine

Laser resurfacing is a new and rapidly improving technique.

wrinkles and sun damage. The laser has solved this problem, and for many patients has eliminated the need for a face-lift.

The photographs on page 152 show a patient before and after ablative laser resurfacing. When laser resurfacing is done correctly on the right person, the results are spectacular. Don't you agree?

But there is a catch: this is surgery, so you'll look terrible for 10–12 days afterwards. You'll have to take meticulous care of your facial skin. In addition, your skin will be red to pink for at least 6 weeks after the surgery. Make-up will make you look fine after about 2 weeks, but don't even think about being seen in public without make-up for at least 6 weeks, possibly longer.

Fortunately, with suitable make-up, you can go back to work and be seen socially by 3 weeks. It is crucial that the appropriate make-up is used. A special 'mineral-based' make-up created by Jane Iredale™ is perfect for the patient who has had laser resurfacing. These superb make-ups can also be used on normal skin.

151

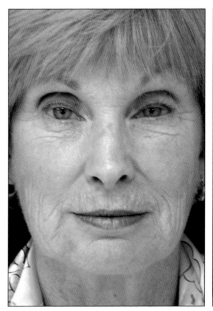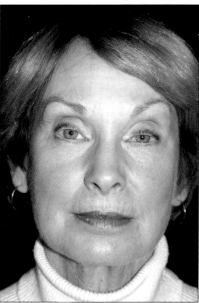

Before (left) and after (right) laser resurfacing.

The final, beautiful result is not complete until 6 months to a year after surgery, but you will be very happy even without make-up from 3 months. Fair-skinned blondes and redheads with wrinkles and sun damage – that is, people with Type I and Type II skin – cannot be given a fresher and younger-looking face by any other means, including a face-lift.

Which laser? The CO_2 laser was the first to be used for laser facial resurfacing[1] and remains the 'gold standard'. However, I also use the erbium laser made by Sciton™, the same scientific brainpower that invented the UltraPulse™ CO_2 laser. The benefit of the erbium laser is that it does not produce as much heat as the CO_2 laser does when it is used on your face. Less heat means less injury, and less injury means faster healing.

Generally, my patients who are treated with the erbium laser heal in one-half to two-thirds the time it takes my CO_2 laser-treated patients to heal. The erbium laser-treated patients are less red for a shorter period of time and ready for make-up earlier. Long term, there is also less chance of hypopigmentation (whitening of the skin or lightening of the laser-treated skin) a year after surgery. However, there are still some situations in which the CO_2 laser is better than the erbium laser, and the decision as to which laser to use requires your doctor to be experienced in laser techniques.

Laser resurfacing is the best facial rejuvenation procedure for the right patient, and the 'right patient' has Type I or Type II skin with very severe wrinkles, sun damage and ageing changes. Nothing else can do as good a job!

Be sure that your doctor shows you pictures of what you will look like 3–4 days and 10 days after the operation. Also, the doctor needs to tell you about potential complications such as infection, scarring, hypopigmentation, prolonged redness and potential eye injury. These complications are rare, and should not happen to you, but they are real risks.

Face-lift

A properly done face-lift, technically called a **rhytidectomy**, can create an elegant, beautifully restored, youthful facial appearance. The face-lift tightens facial skin and removes jowls, tightens the neck and removes the platysmal bands. The brow is elevated and the cheek and malar fat pad are restored to their youthful position over the cheekbone. The nasal–labial fold is tightened and, although the nasal–labial fold line does not disappear, the middle third of the face is freshened significantly. The jaw line is sculpted by a properly done face-lift, and the tired, sometimes angry, look of the aged face is removed. Most commonly, a face-lift is done in conjunction with a blepharoplasty (eyelid rejuvenation), and the result is a nearly total facial rejuvenation that nothing else can match.

After looking at the pictures on page 154, do you *really believe* you can look like that by simply slapping some antioxidant cream on your face? If pills and creams could produce dramatic results like those shown, there would be photographs instead of case histories in the many books touting these therapies. So far, the photographs I have seen showing the results of topical creams and other non-surgical therapies are unimpressive.

If a face-lift is what you need, then have it, but have it performed by a properly trained and accredited plastic surgeon. (I will tell you in the next chapter how to find one.)

What can a face-lift do? It can restore the firmness and integrity of your youthful face, remove jowls and sagging neck, lift the cheek, lift the brow and generally tighten the face.

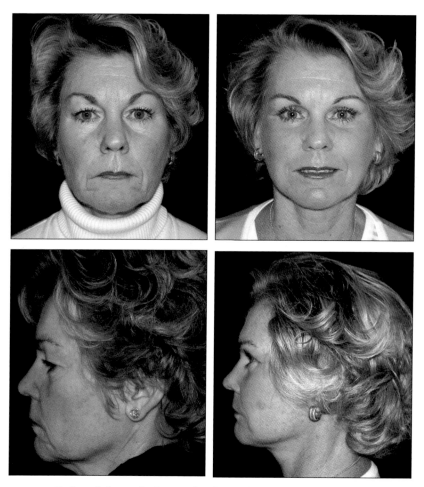

Before (left) and after (right) face-lift and blepharoplasty.

What can a face-lift not do? A face-lift cannot freshen the surface of the skin, remove wrinkles, sun damage, brown spots and dry, hard skin. For that, you need laser resurfacing.

For many patients, the result of a face-lift can be dramatically improved by inserting a chin implant, which gives a beautiful jaw line and youthful neck.

A face-lift firms or tightens loose, sagging facial skin. For fine wrinkles, pigmentation and sun damage, laser resurfacing must be done. Generally, face-lifts are more suitable for darker skin types II, III, IV, V and VI. Face-lifts are often helpful for, and often performed on, patients with Type I or Type II facial skin with severe ageing changes, but these patients usually also need laser resurfacing for the best possible result.

Your age at the time of your face-lift is your business. There are no hard and fast rules. When you see facial sagging in the cheek, the brow, the jaw and the neck, and you are really bothered by these changes, seek a consultation with a reputable, accredited plastic surgeon. It has been my experience that with all restorative and maintenance endeavours, the earlier you repair something that is showing signs of age and wear, the better and longer lasting the repair! I believe the same is true for the face.

A face-lift should not make your face look tight, pulled or unnatural. It should make you look like you did when you were younger. If someone looks like a weasel, this means they either had a bad lift or have had one too many (face-lifts, that is!) Look again at the photographs. These patients simply look younger, not different.

What can go wrong? Potentially, many things, is the short answer. Picking the right surgeon is the key to avoiding problems. Some problems are caused by a failure in a doctor's technique, some are failures in the patient's anatomy and healing, and some are, believe it or not, simply fate.

I show my patients photographs to give them an idea of what they will look like for the first day, a few days later, and 10 days to 2 weeks after surgery. I want them to have no surprises.

Your surgeon should inform you of the possible complications. They are frightening, and they include: bleeding, infection, scarring, skin loss, hair loss, permanent paralysis of the face, loss of feeling in the face, asymmetry or differences in the right and left sides of the face, lumps, bumps and recurrence of sagging. No one can guarantee you a result. Every patient heals differently. One goal is for your result to last 10–15 years, but some patients – generally those with severe sun damage and Type I skin – need a re-do face-lift after 2 years.

In the hands of a skilled, accredited plastic surgeon, *these complications are very rare*. If they were not, we would not be allowed to do this operation. Who would want to? But they can happen, and you need to be informed in advance.

Recovery from a face-lift is usually easier than that from laser resurfacing. The first week after a face-lift your face will be bruised and swollen, although some patients have very little swelling or bruising. Most patients are using make-up by 2 weeks and are back to work by 3 weeks at the latest.

Be wary of the highly marketed mini-face-lift, or weekend tuck. Some patients with minimal facial ageing changes obtain an acceptable result from these less extensive procedures. Many, however, show up in my office needing a revision after having the mini-procedure elsewhere. Of course, the patient ends up paying twice for one final result. As always, it is crucial that you seek expert opinion from a credible source.

Brow-lift

Since the advent of Botox™, which can help elevate the brow, brow-lifting alone is becoming less common. Typically, I perform a **brow-lift** at the same time as I do a face-lift. However, some patients need only a brow-lift. The brow-lift is either done through tiny scalp incisions with an endoscope or with incisions that are hidden in the hairline.

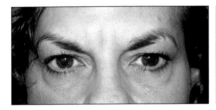 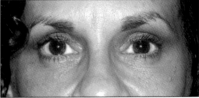

Before (left) and after (right) brow-lift and blepharoplasty.

Complications can include numbness in the forehead, patches of hair loss and recurrence of sagging. Recurrence of brow sagging occurs in about a third of patients. Recovery is much quicker than from a face-lift, usually a week.

Eyelid rejuvenation – blepharoplasty

The eyes are truly the 'windows of the soul', and of all our facial features, they are considered to be the most important. Studies have been carried out on infants who were shown only portions of their mothers' faces – their chins, mouths, noses, foreheads and eyes – and the one part they most frequently and easily recognised was their mothers' eyes.

Unfortunately, as mentioned in Chapter 2, we age first in our eyes, most commonly in our thirties, and some of us in our late twenties. Eyelid rejuvenation is by far the most common plastic surgery operation I perform, and at the earliest age. The results are usually dramatic, pleasing and successful.

Blepharoplasty is intended to correct or partially correct the following ageing changes:

✤ hooding or hanging skin of the upper eyelid,

✤ puffiness (fat herniation of both upper and lower eyelids),

✤ laxity or looseness of the lower eyelid,

✤ tear trough deformity or dark circle (that line under the lower eyelid).

A blepharoplasty alone cannot correct:

✤ brow sagging,

✤ eyelid wrinkles,

✤ ageing damage to eyelid skin,

✤ crow's feet.

Personally, I use the laser for my eyelid rejuvenation procedures. There is less bruising and quicker recovery. Also, I do not make an incision on the outside of the lower eyelid; I use the laser to make an incision on the inside of the lower eyelid, the pink part. This is called a **transconjunctival blepharoplasty**. From the inside of the lower eyelid, I remove or reposition the fat to remove the bulge and partially correct the dark circle. I also use the laser on the inside to shrink or tighten the underlying muscle. Following these manoeuvres, I frequently do what is called a **canthopexy**. The canthopexy is a procedure done through the upper eyelid incision to tighten the tendon of the lower eyelid, recreating the nice curved, upward-slanting lower eyelid appearance of youth.

I often do laser resurfacing on the skin of the lower eyelid to rejuvenate its appearance and remove crow's feet. What's the point of tightening the lower eyelids and removing the bags if the patient still has sun-damaged, aged skin on the eyelid? Patients must go through a period of healing, during which the lower eyelid is red, but when the eyelid has healed and they see brand-new, smooth skin on it, they are very happy.

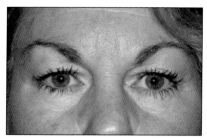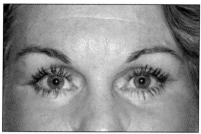

Before (left) and after (right) laser blepharoplasty.

Eyelid wrinkles and crow's feet are also caused by the pulling of the muscle underneath the skin. Therefore, in my practice, I use Botox™ to relax the muscle after surgery, and I encourage patients to continue to have Botox™ treatment of the crow's feet.

The laser is a marvellous, technologically advanced tool that can create optimal results in eyelid rejuvenation. You should find a doctor who is comfortable with and competent in its use, which is not the case for all surgeons.

Complications are rare, but you must be informed: they include bleeding, infection, scarring, dry-eye syndrome (very serious) and ectropion (a sad-eyed or 'hound-dog appearance' that is more common with the external scalpel incision on the lower eyelid – just walk down Rodeo Drive in Beverly Hills or Fifth Avenue in New York and you will see it! Other very rare but serious complications include loss of eyelashes, damage to the eye and even blindness. Your surgeon should discuss them with you.

The above procedures are the most common and effective plastic surgery operations to correct facial ageing. In the next chapter, I will try to help you to make a very important decision if you are considering having plastic surgery.

Reference
1. Seckel, B.R. *Aesthetic Laser Surgery*, 1st edn. Boston: Little, Brown and Company, 1995.

10 Don't let 'just anyone' touch your face!

I am astounded when I hear stories of people who have had potentially dangerous medical and surgical therapies performed by untrained, uncertified people who are not doctors. Recently, in Massachusetts (where I live, and home of the Harvard Medical School and many world-famous doctors and hospitals), police raided a house in one of the suburbs where a man and his wife with no medical training whatsoever were performing blepharoplasty (eyelid surgery) in their home.

I do not know what people are thinking when they subject themselves to such risks, but I do know what they are not thinking. They are not thinking about what they will do when something goes wrong, such as an infection or bleeding. Nor are they thinking about what they will do if the procedure does not produce the result they expect.

There are already significant worries that untrained people without appropriate skills are performing cosmetic facial rejuvenation procedures.[1] More frightening is the fact that there is a proliferation of retail centres, called spas, where nurses and other non-physicians are doing potentially dangerous procedures, supposedly under

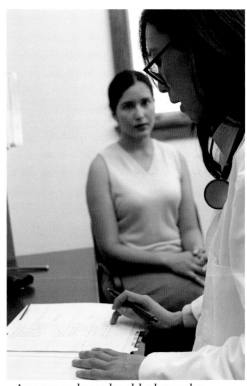

Any procedure should always be performed by a qualified practitioner.

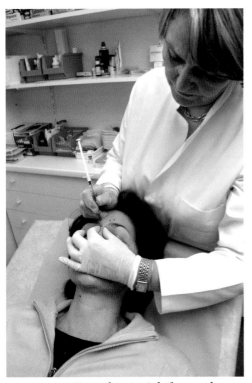

Even for straightforward treatments such as Botox™, you still need a qualified professional.

the supervision of physicians who are not even present at the facility!

I believe a major factor in these occurrences is the perception that cosmetic procedures are simpler than major surgery and therefore less dangerous. Adding to this misconception is the skill and ease with which properly trained physicians perform these procedures, making them look deceptively easy to other physicians and nurses who watch them. In the western United States, a death occurred when a nurse opened her doctor's office at night and performed a liposuction on a friend without the doctor's knowledge. Her friend, the patient, died. I am sure the nurse had watched the doctor do the operation hundreds of times and thought it was simple. Unfortunately, the procedure, which looked so easy when the surgeon was doing it, required skill that can only be learned in a surgical training programme. The nurse accidentally shoved the suction cannula into her friend's liver and the friend bled to death. Do you need to hear more?

Many of the non-surgical procedures performed, such as Botox™ and filler injections, laser treatments and microdermabrasions, are so quick and seemingly easy that you, the patient, do not have the same concern or caution that you would have if you were considering surgery. The problem is, as always, what happens if something goes wrong? What if the Botox™ or the filler is put in the wrong place? How do you set the power of the laser? And how many times do you treat the blood vessel or brown spot?

Money is what is driving these dangerous and misguided practices. Patients want to spend less of it and the non-physician entrepreneurs performing these 'back alley' procedures want to make more of it. Unfortunately, bad things always happen when greed overcomes judgement, principles and ethics.

I hope that, since you are mindful enough to read this book, you will find a qualified physician to advise you and provide or supervise your facial rejuvenation therapies. It is the uninformed people I worry about! So do your part and educate your friends.

So where do you go for advice and treatment for facial rejuvenation? In the UK today, most doctors specialising in facial anti-ageing or facial rejuvenation are plastic surgeons or dermatologists. I am certain there are many others who, as a result of their training, interest and experience, are capable. But the accreditation process in plastic surgery and dermatology provides educational standards that are widely recognised and upheld. Insisting on specialist registration with the General Medical Council (GMC) in one of the above specialties is a good starting place for you, the consumer.

However, consulting an accredited specialist is just the beginning of the process. A certificate on the wall cannot tell you how skilled the doctor is and how expert he or she is in performing facial rejuvenation procedures. There is much more to making an informed decision, as follows.

Be careful – your fear is your friend: how to choose your doctor

Everyone – and I mean everyone – who goes to see a plastic surgeon for the first time is uneasy or fearful. This is a normal self-protective response and you should heed it. Surgery, or any facial procedure, is a very serious undertaking. Essentially, you are giving another person – it is to be hoped, a doctor – control over your facial appearance, your well-being and (in the case of surgery) even your life. This is not something you should take lightly, and most people have inherent, emotional, instinctual responses that **raise a red flag** when they contemplate giving up control of their well-being.

In my experience, there are only two things that can help eliminate your fears, especially when considering the possibility of surgery:

1. complete trust and confidence in your plastic surgeon, or

2. ignorance (sorry for the harsh words, but this is *important*!).

Obviously the second point does not apply to you or you wouldn't be reading this book.

Unfortunately, there are thousands of people who consider having plastic surgery with as much forethought as when they buy a loaf of bread or new blouse. These are the people you see on talk shows condemning plastic surgery because they did not get the results they wanted or, worse, they have been injured. These are tragic, but fortunately rare, occurrences and, like most mistakes we make in life, they could have been avoided.

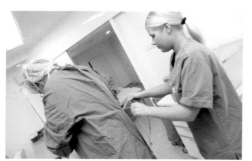

You should feel free to ask any questions you need to about the clinic you choose.

Fortunately, because you're a contemplative and intelligent person, you can undertake the requisite self-education about plastic surgery and learn what you need to know and how to choose a plastic surgeon you can trust to do it right. Knowledge and your 'gut instinct' will lead you to the right person. Remember, 99 per cent of unhappy results are avoidable.

What is a surgeon?

Believe it or not, in the UK today you cannot just assume that a doctor who calls himself or herself a 'surgeon' *is* a surgeon. I am sorry to tell you that some prominent doctors in major metropolitan areas of the UK who openly advertise themselves as 'cosmetic surgeons' have never completed formal surgical training!

There may also be many people who call themselves 'plastic surgeons' who have never had training in an approved plastic surgery training scheme.

How can this be? The simple answer is twofold.

1. We live in a democracy. You can call yourself anything you like. In the USA, the American Society of Plastic and Reconstructive Surgery tried, about 25 years ago, to protect

people from this deception by attempting to prove in court that if you called yourself a plastic surgeon, you should have US board certification and training in plastic surgery. The courts ultimately ruled against the Plastic Surgery Society with a decision that held that to require certification in plastic surgery in order to call oneself a plastic surgeon was a 'restraint of free trade' and violated the Federal Commerce and Communication Act. So much for standards and protections for the consumer! The UK Government and Department of Health take a similar view.

2. There is big money in plastic surgery. Reduced NHS waiting lists and decreasing fees paid by insurance companies have made it more difficult to make a living in private medicine today. There is a widely held misperception that all doctors are wealthy. In fact, most doctors who finished their training in 2005 cannot even think about buying a house until they pay back the debt they acquired obtaining their education.

Aesthetic or cosmetic plastic surgery is the only significant, and growing, 'fee for service' or 'cash and carry field' left in medicine, and it can be very lucrative. Unfortunately, many doctors without formal training or accreditation market themselves as 'cosmetic surgeons' or 'plastic surgeons' because they want to make money and they are not qualified or don't want to undertake the several years of training after medical school that are required to become a fully trained plastic surgeon eligible to be entered on the GMC Specialist Register.

So, dear reader, I have provided you with two of the most important reasons why you should be afraid of letting 'just anyone' touch your unique face. It can be a snake pit out there in certain portions of the non-medical and medical communities, and those of you who simply 'let your fingers do the walking' in the Yellow Pages might as well buy your snake-bite kit and start taking anti-venom now.

In more than 25 years as a plastic surgeon, I have seen some unfortunate complications of plastic surgery performed by unqualified people. When I asked the patients how they found their doctors, the most common answer was – you guessed it – 'in the Yellow Pages'! Another poignant memory is of a woman with terrible scarring who told me, with embarrassment, that her maid had recommended the doctor! Think about it. Do you think the telephone companies ask 'Are you on the specialist register?' before they take £1000 to list someone's advertisement as a plastic surgeon in their book? I doubt it.

So if you can't trust the phone book, or your maid, to help you, how do you find a well-trained, accredited plastic surgeon? Contact the British Association of Aesthetic Plastic Surgeons (www.baaps.org.uk) or the British Association of Plastic, Reconstructive and Aesthetic Surgeons (www.bapras.org.uk) – formerly the British Association of Plastic Surgeons (BAPS). You must be an experienced accredited plastic surgeon to be a full member of these organisations. After you have done your homework and are armed with knowledge, you can start the interview process and evaluate your prospective plastic surgeon. When you have interviewed them, you will then have to listen to the most important protector you have, your 'gut instinct'.

What is an accredited plastic surgeon?

The straightforward, honest answer, and the only answer you should accept, is: a doctor with a medical degree who, after completing medical school, spent 5–7 years in an accredited training programme in one or more fields of surgery, the last 2 years of which were spent in an approved plastic surgery training programme. Doctors must also undergo regular assessment and pass

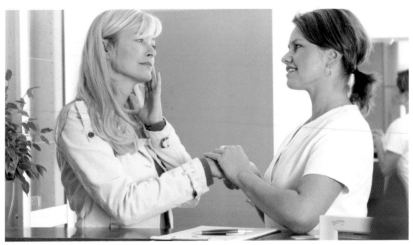

You should feel completely confident in the quality of care you receive.

rigorous written examinations to document that they have an adequate knowledge of the art and science of plastic surgery.

Is this the type of doctor you want to operate on your face? Of course it is. This type of information is not clearly available in the Yellow Pages or newspapers, on the radio or on TV talk shows, on billboards or on the Internet. It is, however, readily available to you, the educated consumer, by contacting the British Association of Aesthetic Plastic Surgeons (www.baaps.org.uk) or the British Association of Plastic, Reconstructive and Aesthetic Surgeons (www.bapras.org.uk). That is how you start your search.

Dermatologists have also made great contributions to the science of facial ageing and have been pioneers in the discovery of skinceuticals, lasers and many of the non-ablative skin treatments discussed earlier in this book. Huge advances in ageing research and breakthroughs in the genetic modification necessary to reverse ageing on the molecular level will probably be made, in part, by dermatologists. They are the skin doctors, and they can do a great deal to help you in your anti-ageing battle. However, they are not surgeons in the sense that they have not trained in surgical training programmes as described earlier.

Most importantly, a fully trained surgeon is trained in how to take care of the whole patient, not just the skin or face, especially if something goes wrong. Furthermore, in my opinion, it takes the 5–7 years of specialised training and experience to learn and understand the complex anatomy and ageing changes that plastic surgery can correct.

There is no recognised surgical subspecialty designated as 'cosmetic surgery'. *Caveat emptor!*

Educate yourself

If you are considering plastic surgery, your general practitioner should refer you to someone whom he or she knows is well trained, ethical and highly skilled. More commonly, happy patients who have had a positive experience with a particular plastic surgeon make plastic surgery 'referrals'. If, however, you do not have the benefit of either of those resources, contact the sources listed above for a referral in your area. I recommend that you get the names of at least two accredited plastic surgeons.

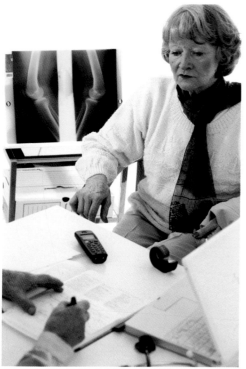

Any reputable plastic surgeon will feel privileged by the trust you place in them.

You are, however, only halfway there. The surgeon you have selected will have to pass another test or oral examination to earn your trust and the privilege and honour of being your doctor.

I sincerely mean that it is an honour and a privilege for a surgeon to have you as a patient. My mentor, and the man who trained me as a plastic surgeon, was Dr Joseph E Murray, Chair of Plastic Surgery at Brigham and Women's Hospital in Boston, Massachusetts, and Professor of Surgery at Harvard Medical School. Dr Murray won the Nobel Prize in Medicine for his work in performing the first kidney transplantation, an event that gave birth to the remarkable field of transplantation surgery. This field has now grown to a level at which kidneys, hearts, lungs, livers, bowels and other essential organs are transplanted, saving lives and preventing disability for thousands of people.

A plastic surgeon started all this? Yes, indeed. Throughout my training and to this day, Dr Murray (now in his eighties) still smiles, eyes glowing, and says, 'I feel so privileged and honoured to be able to be a surgeon,' and he means it. He is the greatest living plastic surgeon and he is honoured and privileged to take care of you.

Every plastic surgeon should feel the same way. You, the patient, are giving us a great honour and privilege by trusting us with your life and well-being. Any surgeon who forgets that and views you as a down payment on a Ferrari or Lamborghini has violated your trust and deserves to be stripped of all credentials and sent packing.

So what can you do to be as certain as possible that the surgeon you have chosen is a person who not only has the education and skills to do a good, safe face-lift or other procedure, but also has the ethical and moral constitution to give you his or her best? Unfortunately, specialist registration and credentials cannot provide you with this insight. Only your instincts and intuition, your 'gut feelings', plus the insights and experiences of other patients who have been treated by the same doctor can help you there. So here's my advice, my recommendations for your consultation.

❀ Do your homework. The British Association of Aesthetic Plastic Surgeons (www.baaps.org.uk) and the British Association of Plastic, Reconstructive and Aesthetic Surgeons (www.bapras.org.uk) provide easy-to-understand information about all cosmetic surgery. You can call them or go to their websites and receive educational brochures about any procedure you are interested in. Do this and read about the surgery you are considering.

❀ Write down your questions ahead of your consultation. Be prepared. If you have knowledge, you have power. You must know what to ask your surgeon. Ask the right questions. Here are a few questions that may not be in the brochures.

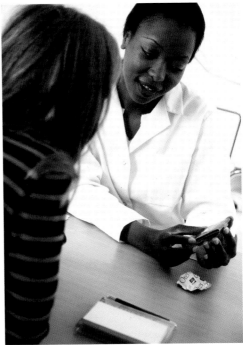

1. Are you on the GMC Specialist Register for Plastic Surgery? Get a straight answer here; merely being registered with the GMC (a statement commonly used by those NOT on the Specialist Register and probably intended to mislead you) is a requirement of all practising doctors in the UK and implies no special training past medical school!

Your surgeon will be happy to answer your questions.

2. Are you experienced in or do you specialise in aesthetic and cosmetic plastic surgery? This is important, I believe. Many superb reconstructive plastic surgeons have little experience in cosmetic plastic surgery. You must ask the question.

3. How many of these operations have you done? Do you do them frequently?

4. Are you comfortable operating on me? Do you think that this operation is appropriate for me? We are all very different, with specific, challenging anatomical issues.

5. What can go wrong? What are the possible complications? How often do they occur?

6. What happens if something goes wrong? Is a revision or correction free of charge or will I have to pay for it?

7. On how many visits or how many times after surgery do I get to see you? Can I reach you or someone with access to you 24/7 after my surgery? Is someone available to see me nights, weekends or holidays if I have a problem?

8. Will you allow me to contact and talk with patients you have operated on who can tell me what their experiences have been?

These are excellent questions to ask and you have every right to expect clear, honest answers. They reflect that you have done your homework and are an educated patient. Believe me, a good surgeon will be grateful that you are prepared, as patients who are unprepared and lack the necessary knowledge can cause problems after surgery. However, ensure that your information comes from reliable sources. The Internet is unregulated and much of the information to be found on it is either incorrect or even deliberately misleading. Remember that much Internet content is advertising only.

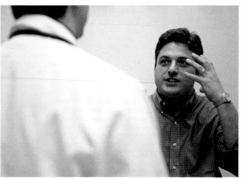

Trust your instincts. If you don't feel comfortable with the surgeon, just leave.

I try very hard to inform my patients before surgery of what to expect, and we give our patients 'informed consent' forms that are legally prepared documents outlining the possible complications and problems. Research has shown that patients forget 90 per cent of what they are told and what they have confirmed by their signatures that they have read and understood. This is a very difficult problem. It may be hard, but you, the patient, need to do your part and be an educated consumer.

Trust your 'gut feelings' and 'red flags'

Here, I am stating what should seem to be the obvious, but how many times in our lives do we have that 'gut feeling', ignore it, make a decision and regret it? Having plastic surgery is not like buying a car, an expensive diamond or a £10,000 gown. Any of those things can be a bad choice that costs you money and puts you in debt, but you are still alive and well afterwards! Your friends can still recognise you and you can learn from your mistake and restore your life.

Choosing the wrong person to do plastic surgery on your face could result in irreversible deformity and loss of your health and/or self-esteem and turn your happiest dreams into a nightmare.

I don't want to dissuade you. Many thousands of people have superb plastic surgery every year in this country and complications are very, very rare when the right operation is done on the right patient by the right surgeon. I want the best for you and I want you to have a good experience. If you do, you will bring happiness to yourself and honour to my profession. But there are a few things, which I call 'red flags', that are warnings from your intuitive self that are trying to protect you. Listen to them.

❀ First, remind yourself that the doctor you are seeing wants you as a patient. Cosmetic surgery is elective surgery, and you are paying cash for your operation. *You* are doing the favour here. The doctor should be kind, warm, concerned and respectful of you as a person. If he or she doesn't make you feel this way, then smile politely, say, 'Thank you. I will get back to you when I make my decision,' and leave. The most important question to ask yourself is, 'Do I trust this person? Will I feel comfortable having this person take care of me if something goes wrong?' If the answer is no, leave. Do you remember what

169

Jenny said in the movie *Forrest Gump* when the mean boys were chasing him? She yelled, 'Run, Forrest, run!'

✿ The surgeon is cold. This one should be a no-brainer. It's not your problem if the surgeon's parents weren't nurturing enough or if this person's life has been tough. Some of our greatest geniuses (think Mozart) are driven to achieve great skills by their tormented souls. Years of training, scrutiny and rigorous testing cannot guarantee basic human compassion and kindness. Trust your feelings. Talk to the doctor. Look in his/her eyes and face. Would you be comfortable asking this person to help you when you are frightened, in need, even with your silliest question? You should be. If you are not, 'Run, Forrest, run!'

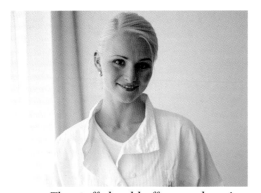

The staff should offer a welcoming and professional atmosphere.

✿ The surgeon becomes uncomfortable, defensive or angry when you ask those important questions that you must ask. Again, trust your instincts. He or she should welcome your questions and answer them to your satisfaction. If you see sweat on the surgeon's brow or the initial warm glow of your meeting disappears, 'Run, Forrest, run!'

✿ The surgeon does not act like a doctor. Personally, I like a white coat or a conservative suit or dress. Even casual relaxed is okay. I frequently wear scrubs and a white coat in my office. If your surgeon acts like a used-car salesman or looks like he or she is dressed to go onstage in Las Vegas, I would get nervous. The surgeon's professionalism and credentials are what is important here, not the authentic Ming vase in the waiting room. Don't get me wrong; I love Ming vases (wish I could afford one) and pretty things. I believe, and it is my practice in my office, that the plastic surgery office should be appointed and designed for your comfort and enjoyment. But if you are more awed by the decor and the trappings than by the professionalism of the surgeon, 'Run, Forrest, run!'

❧ The surgeon or the staff makes you feel stupid for asking a question. Come on now, you wouldn't be reading this book if you didn't already know that game. Do you like or trust or want to be around anyone who makes you feel less than you truly are, which is a worthwhile human being with normal concerns, anxieties and fear? You are coming to a professional whose job it is to make you feel good about yourself. If you do not, 'Run, Forrest, run!'

❧ If it seems too good to be true, it is. C'mon, you know this. If this thought pops in your mind, respect it, 'Run, Forrest, run!'

❧ Plastic surgery is not cheap. Surgery includes the skills and training of your surgeon and very high-tech, expensive equipment, anaesthesia, nursing and complex postoperative care. Any plastic surgeon who offers you a cut-rate deal is leaving out something important, and when it comes to your health and safety, you cannot afford to leave anything out. This includes the offer of free consultation, and other 'offers'. In the USA, the American Society for Aesthetic Plastic Surgery publishes average fees for various cosmetic procedures, but there is no equivalent list of prices in the UK. So simply ask your surgeon how his or her fee compares to the national average. Yes, it is cheaper in a clinic than in a hospital, but is it a safe clinic? Ask where you would be taken if something goes wrong. In plastic surgery, I would be less worried if a surgeon charges more than the average. There is usually a good reason: they are the best, and their expertise and reputation permit them to charge more. Whether they are really worth it can be ascertained when you speak with patients who have had operations performed by that surgeon. Be sure to ask for permission to talk with previous patients. If someone offers you a bargain or a cut rate, 'Run, Forrest, run!'

❧ The plastic surgeon's staff – the receptionist and nurses, and possibly also assistant, technicians, physician assistants and medical aestheticians – play a crucial role in your experience. They will have a significant role in your postoperative care and will be invaluable to you. Talk with them and trust your instincts. Are they professional, warm, kind, caring people you would be comfortable asking for help and depending on? Don't choose them because they are physically attractive, well-dressed starlets! They are health-care professionals, not models. If you feel as though you do not belong there, you most certainly do not. 'Run, Forrest, run!'

❧ Choose a plastic surgeon who performs cosmetic surgery regularly. Plastic surgery not only involves knowledge and judgement but, as surgery, also requires manual skills and dexterity. Those who don't have them are typically weeded out during training. However, whether you are playing a piano, painting a house, doing a cross-stitch or performing plastic surgery, *practice makes perfect*. The British Association of Aesthetic Plastic Surgeons is a society of plastic surgeons who have a special interest and expertise in cosmetic plastic surgery. Their website (www.baaps.org.uk) has detailed information about all cosmetic procedures and is an excellent place for you to learn about the procedure you are considering. Ask the surgeon whether he or she does cosmetic surgery regularly and, if the response makes you feel anxious, 'Run, Forrest, run!'

Finally, in deference to my younger colleagues, let me say that old and experienced is not necessarily better than young and skilled. Grey hair is no guarantee. There are many brilliant, young, accredited plastic surgeons who are better educated, trained and skilled than ever before. They can do as good a job, or even better, than an older, less-talented surgeon. It's a balance. You need to ask the right questions and trust your instincts – your 'gut feelings'. And remember, try to talk to prior patients.

Plastic surgery addiction – body dysmorphic disorder

In my experience, most patients seeking facial rejuvenation treatments and plastic surgery are sensitive, wonderful, sane, well-adjusted individuals who consider looking their best to be one part of an overall positive attitude towards life and health. There are, however, some people who seek plastic surgery not simply to fight ageing and improve the way they look, but rather to correct some imagined deformity that only they can see. This type of patient is more likely to be young and there is evidence that this phenomenon is more common in males.

All ethical, well-trained, accredited plastic surgeons should be aware of this disorder, called **body dysmorphic disorder**, and encourage these individuals to seek psychiatric care, not surgery. However, as mentioned earlier in this chapter, there are some unscrupulous, inadequately trained, non-medical and medical practitioners who are more concerned about making money than they are about the health and welfare of their patients. Often, patients who have been turned down by reputable plastic surgeons end up having their surgery in these 'back alley' practices, frequently with disastrous results.

The media refers to people who have had too many plastic surgery procedures as 'plastic surgery addicts'. However, body dysmorphic disorder is the proper medical terminology for a serious, painful, distressing obsession with imagined physical deformity. When you see people with this disorder, you usually cannot imagine what they find unappealing about their appearance! Individuals afflicted with this illness go to incredible behavioural extremes to modify their appearance. I am not talking about three or four plastic surgeries, but ten or twenty!

Obviously, the doctor has to avoid operating on these individuals. However, patients are not always honest and forthcoming about their medical histories and it is possible for a well-meaning doctor to be misled and to operate on someone without being fully aware of his or her motivation for surgery.

Body dysmorphic disorder is defined as follows.[2]

❦ Preoccupation with some imagined defect in appearance. If a slight physical anomaly is present, the person's concern is markedly excessive.

❦ The preoccupation causes clinically significant distress or impairment in social, occupational or other important areas of functioning.

❦ The preoccupation is not better accounted for by another mental disorder (e.g. dissatisfaction with body shape and size in anorexia nervosa).

The above definition does not describe an individual who is a 'little vain'; rather, it characterises someone with a serious obsessive disorder. If the above description applies to you, a friend or someone you love, I urge you to read or refer the involved person to

The Broken Mirror by Katharine A. Phillips, MD.[2] There are clinics at the Maudsley Hospital and the Priory Hospital in London, and an informative website at www.bddcentral.com.

Keep up to date

The field of anti-ageing medicine generally, and facial rejuvenation in particular, is advancing rapidly. New information and therapies are discovered almost daily, and it is crucial that you continue to read and inform yourself. I hope this book has stimulated you to educate yourself further about staying healthy and safe and looking and feeling your best. As new research and technologies evolve, I will attempt to keep this information updated on my website, www.saveyourface.com.

My goal in writing this book has been to teach you the truth about this important and increasingly popular topic. I have tried to provide a balanced and honest presentation that includes the risks as well as the rewards of pursuing some form of facial rejuvenation as part of an overall programme of health and self-improvement. Obviously, as a plastic surgeon, I believe in the value and worth of my profession, and sincerely hope that what you have learned in this book will help you safely and happily achieve your goals.

Good luck and good health! It is my hope that we will be able to continue this important discussion and our relationship through cyberspace.

References

1. Hubbs, L. Treating complications caused by non-physicians. *Skin & Ageing* 10:57, 2002.
2. Phillips, K.A. *The Broken Mirror: Understanding and Treating Body Dysmorphic Disorder.*
New York: Oxford University Press, 1986.

Glossary

Ablative Referring to a procedure that involves the cutting off or removal of cells from the surface of the skin.

Accredited plastic surgeon A doctor with a medical degree and 5–7 years in an accredited surgical training programme, including at least 2 in an approved plastic surgery programme.

Acne A group of skin rashes with various causes.

Actinic keratoses Dry, scaling, patches of irritated skin (keratoses) caused by sun (actinic) damage to the skin. May be a precursor to skin cancer.

Aesthetician A licensed professional who recommends and practises skin care and the use of treatments for beauty and health.

Age spots Pigmented (brown) spots on the skin seen in older people. Also called 'liver spots' and 'sun spots'. They are most common on the hands and face, the areas most frequently exposed to the sun, and represent the skin's attempt to protect itself from the sun by producing pigment.

Allergenic Referring to any substance that causes hypersensitivity or an allergic reaction.

Allergic reaction The hypersensitive response of the immune system to a substance to which an individual is allergic.

Alternative medicine A wide range of healing methods not used in conventional Western medicine. Also described as 'complementary medicine'.

American Board of Plastic Surgery An organisation that oversees and implements the board-certification process in plastic surgery in the USA.

American Council on Graduate Medical Education (ACGME) The organisation that oversees and regulates the residency training programmes of the various medical and surgical specialties in the USA.

American Society for Aesthetic Plastic Surgery A society of US board-certified plastic surgeons with special interest and experience in aesthetic or cosmetic plastic surgery.

American Society of Plastic Surgeons A society of US board-certified plastic surgeons that sponsors continuing education in plastic surgery and the enforcement of ethical and professional standards. Board certification in plastic surgery is required for membership.

Andropause A phenomenon similar to the female menopause that occurs in men and is related to a fall in levels of the hormone testosterone.

Antioxidant Any compound or element that prevents oxidation by free radicals.

Antioxidant vitamins Vitamins that prevent oxidation by scavenging or removing free radicals.

Arachidonic acid A omega-6 fatty acid that is present in cell membranes and released when they are damaged.

Atom The smallest unit into which matter can be divided and still retain the characteristic properties of the element.

Atrophy Wasting away.

Autoimmune response A response of the body's immune system in which its defence system attacks the host body. Rheumatoid arthritis is an example.

Basal cell carcinoma A skin cancer arising in the basal layer (the deep layer) of the epithelium. It is more common in sun-exposed areas of the body, and in people with less genetically determined sun protection, i.e. fair-skinned individuals.

Bleaching agents Topical solutions that bleach or lighten brown pigmented areas when applied to the skin.

Blepharoplasty A plastic surgical operation performed on the eyelids to remove excess skin and fat in order to restore a youthful appearance to the eyelids. Also known as an 'eyelid tuck'.

Board-certified physician A US physician who has successfully completed an approved residency training programme and a certifying examination in a medical or surgical specialty approved by the American Council on Graduate Medical Education (ACGME).

Body dysmorphic disorder A psychological illness characterised by an obsessive preoccupation with an imagined physical defect.

Botox" A purified protein derived from a toxin produced by the bacterium *Clostridium botulinum*. It works by preventing nerve impulses from reaching a muscle, causing the muscle to relax, and can be used to paralyse a muscle temporarily to reduce or eliminate wrinkles or frown lines.

British Association of Aesthetic Plastic Surgeons The association set up to advance education about, and the practice of, plastic surgery in the UK.

British Association of Plastic, Reconstructive and Aesthetic Plastic Surgeons A professional representative body for plastic surgeons in the UK.

Brow ptosis Sagging of the eyebrow.

Brow-lift A plastic surgical operation to lift the brow and restore a youthful appearance to the forehead and eyes.

Brown spots Brown or pigmented spots on the skin caused by sun exposure and ageing. Also called 'age spots', 'liver spots' and 'sun spots'.

Bunny lines Wrinkles around the base of the nose between the eyes caused by the pull of the muscles of facial expression.

Canthopexy A surgical procedure to tighten the lower eyelid by shortening the supporting structures at the lateral canthal tendon.

Cell The smallest structural unit of living matter that is able to function independently.

Cell membrane A thin layer that forms the outer boundary of a living cell.

Chemical peel A procedure in which an irritant such as an acid is applied to the skin to remove the outer layers of skin cells and injure the deeper layers of the skin to stimulate new collagen production.

Chromosome A thread-like strand of DNA and associated proteins in the nucleus of cells that carries the genes.

Collagen A fibrous structural protein produced by fibroblasts in the dermis of the skin and also present in bone, cartilage, tendon and other connective tissue.

Coronary artery disease The accumulation of fat-laden plaques within the walls of the blood vessels in the heart, which interrupt blood flow to the heart muscle and cause 'heart attacks'.

Cortisol A hormone produced by the adrenal gland in response to stress. Elevated levels increase the heart rate and have a profound ageing effect on the cells of the face and body.

Cosmetologist An expert in the use of cosmetics.

Crow's feet Lines around the outside corners of the eyelids that form during facial ageing. They are caused by the pull of the muscles of facial expression.

Cruciferous vegetables Vegetables with thick, partially developed flower structures and fleshy stalks, rich in antioxidant vitamins, e.g. broccoli and cauliflower.

Cytokines Chemical messengers released in the body after injury to a cell. They signal the elements from the bloodstream to initiate the inflammatory response.

Dark circles Shadows under the lower eyelid caused by ageing changes beneath the skin. Frequently described as a 'tired look'.

Dermaplaning The mechanical removal of dead skin from the face using a scalpel.

Dermatologist A doctor who specialises in skin diseases.

Dermis The deep layer of the skin below the epidermis, and the location of the collagen and elastin necessary for skin elasticity.

Detoxification The process by which toxins are removed from the body, and in which the liver plays a primary role.

Digestive enzyme deficiency A condition in which inadequate digestion of food results in partially digested food acting as a foreign protein and stimulating an immune response.

DNA (Deoxyribonucleic acid) A complex organic compound found in all living cells and viruses; the substance which makes up genes.

Down time The time required for recovery following a surgical procedure.

Dynamic wrinkles Wrinkles that are visible when the face is moving – frown lines, laugh lines, worry lines and crow's feet. They are caused by the pull of the facial muscles beneath the skin and may eventually become static wrinkles.

Eczema An inflammatory skin disorder characterised by itching, scaling and thickening of the skin. It is most common on the face, elbows, knees and arms.

Elasticity The ability of the skin to return to its original shape after being pulled or stretched.

Elastin A specialised form of collagen found in the dermis that is responsible for the elasticity of the skin.

Electron The lightest sub-atomic particle known. It carries a negative (–) electrical charge.

Endocrinologist A doctor who specialises in treating disorders of the hormone-secreting endocrine glands, e.g. diabetes.

Epidermis The outer surface layer of the skin.

Epithelial cells The skin cells that make up the epidermis.

Erbium laser A laser with a wavelength of 2.94 microns used for facial resurfacing.

Exfoliation The process of removing the outer, usually dead, layers of the skin.

Extrinsic ageing Ageing changes that are precipitated or caused by factors outside the body.

Eyelid bags Puffiness or fullness of the lower eyelids caused by the pressure of protruding fat beneath the skin.

Face-lift A plastic surgical operation to tighten or lift the facial skin and restore a youthful appearance to the face.

Facial rejuvenation The process of restoring a face to a more youthful form and appearance.

Fat transplantation A plastic surgical procedure in which fat cells are removed from one area of the body and surgically placed into another area. This procedure is most commonly performed to fill depressions or lines in the face caused by ageing.

Fibroblast A specialised cell in the body that has the ability to produce or manufacture collagen. This cell is the primary cell in the process of scar formation.

Fibrosis The production of excess collagen by the fibroblasts in response to inflammation, which results in the formation of a scar.

Fillers Synthetic or manufactured substances that are injected into the skin to 'plump up' or fill depressions or wrinkles in the skin caused by ageing.

Fractional photothermolysis A process used in Fraxel™ laser treatment by which the laser beam is broken up into tiny beams that spread out and ablate microscopic treatment zones beneath the skin's surface, leaving the surrounding skin intact.

Free radical A molecule containing at least one unpaired electron (–). Free radicals can cause significant damage to the cells of the body. They are produced during the metabolism of food in the mitochondria.

Free-radical scavengers Substances that attach to, and render harmless, free radicals, for example vitamin C and other antioxidant vitamins.

Frown lines Lines between the eyebrows that are accentuated during frowning and become permanent with ageing. They are caused by the pull of the muscles of facial expression.

Gene A structure composed of DNA that resides on the chromosomes in the nucleus of the cell and determines heredity. Genes exert their influence by controlling the molecular machinery of the cell.

Glycation The attachment of a glucose or sugar molecule to a protein, creating damage and rendering the protein ineffective.

Heart attack Damage to the muscle of the heart caused by interruption of the blood flow to the heart. The classic symptom is chest pain. A heart attack can be fatal.

Herniate To rupture or push through.

Histamine A chemical released by the mast cell during an inflammatory response. The response of the body to histamine release is dilatation of the blood vessels, which causes redness of the skin, watering of the eyes and runny nose, often called an allergic response.

Hormone replacement therapy (HRT) Therapy to replace the hormone oestrogen after menopause.

Human Genome Project A research project designed to map and identify the genes located on the human chromosome. The identification of the structure of the human genes will enable scientists to synthesise genes and insert them into abnormal cells to correct genetic abnormalities that cause diseases such as diabetes.

Human growth hormone A hormone responsible for growth and development in the human. Levels decrease with age, and correction of deficiencies of this hormone have been associated with remarkable anti-ageing effects.

Hyaluronic acid A biologically active compound called a mucopolysaccharide found in all tissues but in highest concentrations in the embryo. It is present in the skin and is responsible for moisture content. It decreases dramatically with ageing.

Hyperpigmentation Darkening of the skin, particularly of the face and other areas commonly exposed to sunlight, which occurs in the form of brown spots or patches. It is most often the result of ultraviolet radiation stimulating the production of the brown pigment melanin in the melanocytes of the skin.

Hypopigmentation Spots or patches of light skin colour that can occur following laser treatment.

Inflammation A response of the cells of the body to injury that releases histamine and ultimately leads to proliferation of fibroblasts and scarring.

Infomercials Advertisements that purport to be providing impartial educational information but in reality are commercials designed to stimulate people to buy a product.

Infrared Light with a wavelength of 0.7–10.6 microns emitted by heat, used for night vision equipment and as an energy source for collagen remodelling.

Insulin A hormone released by the pancreas that is essential for the breakdown of starches, the entrance of carbohydrates into the bloodstream, and the metabolism of sugars and fats.

Intense pulsed light (IPL) Light generated by a flash lamp in a machine through a lens designed to allow through specific therapeutic wavelengths of light used to remove pigment and blood vessels and to stimulate new collagen production in the skin.

Intestinal dysbiosis The imbalance of the normal bacterial flora present in the large intestine caused by the consumption of antibiotics, both prescription and in the food supply.

Intrinsic ageing Ageing of the body caused by internal or inherent factors.

Jowls Sagging of the lower cheek area at the jawline of the face that can occur as the skin of the face descends with ageing.

Laser A machine designed to produce an intense beam of light that is monochromatic (one colour) and coherent (stays together). Laser stands for **l**ight **a**mplification by **s**timulated **e**mission of **r**adiation. Energy, usually electrical, is supplied to a tube containing a gas. The electrical energy forces electrons away from the atoms of the gas in the tube; the electrons are accelerated by bouncing off mirrors in the tube and are released from the tube as powerful light beams.

Laser resurfacing A plastic surgical procedure during which a laser beam is used to ablate (remove) old damaged skin from the face and injure the dermis so that new skin, new epithelium and new dermis, with new dermal collagen is formed, and wrinkles and sun damage are removed.

Light-emitting diode (LED) The red blinking light you see on your remote control and microwave.

Linoleic acid A polyunsaturated fatty acid that is a major constituent in many vegetable oils. It is used by the body in the synthesis of prostaglandins and cell membranes and helps prevent skin dryness and roughness. However, high levels in the body convert to arachidonic acid, which is toxic.

Lipstick lines Vertical lines in the skin around the lips caused by the pull of the muscles of facial expression, which are more noticeable with ageing and heavily accentuated by smoking cigarettes.

Loss of elasticity A failure of the skin to return to its normal shape after being pulled or stretched.

Low-density lipoprotein (LDL) cholesterol The major cholesterol carrier in the blood. If too much LDL cholesterol circulates in the blood, it can slowly build up in the walls of the arteries feeding the heart and brain. It is also referred to as 'bad' cholesterol.

Macrophage A cell that responds to inflammation by migrating into the injured area and ingesting and removing damaged cells. Once the damaged cells have been removed, the macrophage transforms into a fibroblast and produces collagen and a scar.

Malar fat pad A pad of fat high in the cheek on top of the cheekbone in youth, which is responsible for the 'chubby cheeks' of children. With facial ageing and loss of elasticity, the fat pad falls, creating a hollow where it used to be. The hollow contributes to the tear trough deformity.

Marionette lines Deep lines below the corners of the mouth caused by sagging of the cheek skin with ageing of the face.

Mast cell A cell involved in the initiation of the inflammatory response. Following injury, mast cells migrate into the injured area and release chemicals such as histamine that begin the inflammatory response.

Melanoma A malignant form of skin cancer arising from the pigment cells of the skin. Intense sun exposure, especially to fair-skinned children, increases the risk of this cancer in later life.

Melatonin A hormone secreted by the pineal gland in the brain that controls sleep/wake cycles. This hormone is believed by some to have anti-ageing properties.

Menopause The final cessation of menstruation, ending female fertility.

MicroLaserPeel" A superficial type of laser skin peel performed with the erbium laser. The depth of this skin peel is usually 20–40 microns.

Microdermabrasion A 'no down time' skin peel performed by superficially abrading the skin using a device that passes silica particles across skin while it is held tight to the device by vacuum pressure. The depth of the peel is usually 8 microns.

MicroPeel" A superficial skin peel performed by mechanically scraping dead skin off the face using a scalpel, a technique called dermaplaning. After dermaplaning, a dilute solution of alpha-hydroxy acids is applied to the skin. The depth of the procedure is approximately 5 microns.

Micron A unit of measurement that is one-thousandth of a millimetre (one-millionth of a metre).

Mitochondria [singular: mitochondrion] A small structure in the cytoplasm of the cell that is responsible for the production of energy from the metabolism of food. Free radicals are generated during this process.

Molecule The smallest particle of a substance that retains all the properties of the substance and is composed of one or more atoms.

Muscles of facial expression The muscles of the face responsible for facial expression during acts such as smiling, frowning, crying, etc. With facial ageing, the pull of these muscles creates wrinkles or lines on the face, called the lines of facial expression.

Nasal–labial fold A fold of cheek skin hanging over a line that runs from the outside corner of the nostril to the corner of the mouth.

Nasal–labial fold line The line beneath the nasal–labial fold caused by the pull of the smile muscles.

'No down time' procedure The term used in this book to refer to facial rejuvenation procedures that produce minimal or no redness or discomfort and do not require a recovery period. Thus a person may have this type of procedure and return to work or other normal daily activity immediately.

Non-ablative therapy The term used in this book to describe a facial rejuvenation therapy that does not ablate (remove) the superficial layer of the skin (the epidermis) and thus does not create an open wound that would require postoperative care.

Oestrogen A class of sex hormone that primarily affects the development, maturation and function of the female reproductive system.

pH A measure of the acidity of a solution: pH 7 is neutral; an acidic solution has a pH below 7; and an alkaline solution has a pH above 7.

Pigment cells Cells of the skin that produce pigment, or colour; also called melanocytes. These cells are responsible for skin colour, tanning, brown spots, age spots and sunspots.

Plastic surgeon A surgeon certified by the BAAPS or BAPRAS.

Plastic surgery A surgical specialty that involves the reconstruction of the face and other body tissues to correct defects in appearance or restore function.

Plastic surgery addiction A lay term used to describe body dysmorphic disorder, a condition manifested by a person having multiple plastic surgeries to correct an imagined or minor physical deformity.

Platysmal band A band or fold of skin hanging below the chin, running from the chin down into the neck.

Processed foods Foods that have been altered from their natural form by chemical or mechanical manipulation or the addition of preservatives or other compounds.

Prostaglandins A group of hormone-like fatty acid compounds that have many effects throughout the body, including in inflammation, smooth muscle contraction and regulating body temperature, and on certain hormones. They are made by skin cells from fats in the diet, and help keep the skin soft and smooth.

Proton A particle that is identical to the nucleus of the hydrogen atom, and that, together with neutrons, is a constituent of all other atomic nuclei. It carries a positive charge numerically equal to the charge of an electron.

Psoriasis A chronic disease of the skin marked by inflamed, red patches covered with white scales.

Radiofrequency Radiant energy of a certain frequency, greater than 10 microns and up to thousands of metres. It is used to transmit radio and television, but also in specialised machines to tighten skin.

Raise a red flag A warning, usually of impending danger; for example, red flags are raised in coastal areas to warn of an approaching hurricane.

Refined starches Carbohydrates such as sugar and flour that have been chemically or mechanically altered or processed to change them from their natural state.

Retin-A" A retinoid used as a topical skin solution to stimulate new cell formation by the epidermis and the production of new collagen in the dermis.

Retinoids A class of topical skin drugs, derived from vitamin A, used for treating acne, psoriasis, sun damage and facial ageing. These drugs are keratolytic, which means that they remove keratin, the compound contained in superficial skin cells.

Retinols Retinoids that are precursors to tretinoin (Retin-A"). They are not as powerful as tretinoin and can be used in patients with sensitive skin.

Rhytidectomy The medical term for a face-lift. *Rhytid* means loose skin; *ectomy* means to cut out or remove.

Rosacea A skin disorder manifested by a pink or red flush and dilated blood vessels in the skin of the face around the nose and on the cheeks.

Scar Fibrous tissue replacing normal tissue as a result of injury or disease.

Sebum An oily substance produced by the sebaceous glands in the skin that is a mixture of fat and the debris of dead fat-producing cells.

Skin cancer A cancer arising in the skin.

Skin laxity Looseness of the skin caused by loss of elasticity.

Skin peel A procedure during which the outer layers of the skin are removed or peeled away, usually by the application of an acid or a laser.

Skin type The genetically determined characteristics of skin, including its colour, thickness and susceptibility to sunburn, and associated with characteristic hair and eye colour.

Skinceuticals A term used to refer to topical solutions applied to the skin for the purpose of exerting a pharmacological effect, also called cosmaceuticals.

Smile lines Lines around the mouth and on the cheeks created during the act of smiling.

Solar elastosis A pathological diagnosis made on microscopic examination of the skin and manifested by the accumulation of damaged elastin fibres in the deeper layers of the dermis. This condition is caused by damage to the dermal collagen and elastin by the ultraviolet rays of the sun and by ageing.

Squamous cell carcinoma A skin cancer consisting of the epithelial cells of the skin.

Static wrinkles Wrinkles that are present in the skin when the face is at rest and that are caused by the loss of collagen in the deeper layers of the skin.

Statin drugs Drugs used to lower blood cholesterol.

Stroke A medical illness caused by loss of blood supply to the brain, which can result in paralysis, other neurological symptoms or death.

Sun-damaged skin Skin that has been damaged by long-term exposure to the sun, which results in wrinkles, brown spots, actinic keratoses and dry skin.

Supratarsal fold A curved line on the upper eyelid that appears between 8 and 12 millimetres above the eyelashes.

Target-specific photothermolysis The destruction of a specific target by heat produced by light energy, most commonly a laser.

Tear trough deformity A line or trough running from the corner of the eye near the nose down and out to the side of the face across the cheek.

Telangiectasia A collection of small dilated blood vessels that appear as a red spot on the skin, most commonly around the nose and on the cheek and chin.

Telomerase An enzyme that mediates the repair of the telomere.

Telomere The end portion of a chromosome that controls the number of times a cell can divide.

Testosterone The most potent naturally occurring male or androgenic sex hormone, which is produced primarily by the testes and affects the development, maturation and function of the male reproductive system.

Thyroid hormone A hormone produced by the thyroid gland that has profound effects on the metabolic rate of the body.

Time urgency Having too much to do in too little time.

Topical agents Medications applied directly to the skin, as opposed to those taken internally by mouth.

Transconjunctival blepharoplasty An eyelid rejuvenation operation performed through a small incision inside the eyelid so that there is no visible scar left on the outside of the eyelid skin.

Turkey wattle Loose folds of skin on the neck below the chin that are caused by the skin becoming lax as it ages.

Ultraviolet (UV) light Light with a wavelength less than 0.4 microns, which occupies from violet on the visible light spectrum down to the X-ray portion of the electromagnetic spectrum. Ultraviolet radiation comes from sunlight and is divided into three bands: UVA, UVB and UVC (which does not reach the Earth). UVB has the most profound effect on the skin, causing sunburn, ageing changes and skin cancer. UVA has similar but less intense damaging effects on the skin.

Vitamin One of a group of organic substances present in minute amounts in natural foodstuffs that are essential to normal metabolism. Significant deficiencies of some vitamins can cause serious medical illness.

Worry lines Transverse lines that run across the forehead, accentuated by the facial expression associated with worry or stress. They are caused by the pull of the muscles of facial expression.

Wrinkle As used in this book, a linear depression or crease in the skin associated with ageing, particularly when present in the facial skin. Factors that contribute to the formation of wrinkles in the skin are damage to and atrophy of the collagen and elastin in the dermis, loss of skin elasticity, atrophy of subcutaneous fat, and the pull of the muscles of facial expression.

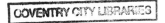

Index

Page numbers in *italics* indicate illustrations; those in **bold** indicate major references